# AFLATOXIN IN CATTLE FEED, MILK AND POSSIBLE CONTROL

## *The Authors*

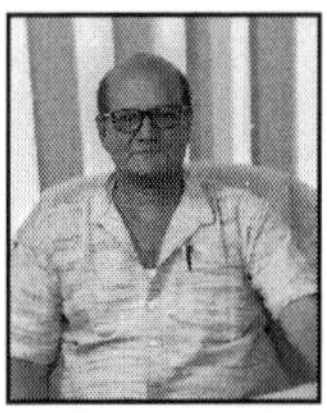

**Dr. Ajoy Kumar Choudhary** is Senior Associate Professor at University Dept. of Botany. He did his Ph.D. and Post Doctoral Fellowship under the supervision of Late Prof. (Dr.) K.S. Bilgrami, FNA. Dr. Choudhary is the recipient of Jawaharlal Nehru Award (I.C.A.R.) in 1995 for Best Ph.D Thesis in India (Plant Protection) and U.G.C Post Doctoral Research Award (2004). Dr. Choudhary has published more than four dozen research papers in Journals of International reputes.

Dr. Choudhary has administrative experiences of more than 10 years as Course Co-ordinator/ Director U.G (TNB College) and P.G Dept. of Biotechnology, TMBU. He has completed more than 08 Research Projects of UGC and DEFCC, Govt. of Bihar on various aspects of mycotoxicology and plant tissue culture technology. Dr. Choudhary is the nominated expert resource person of State Bamboo Mission, Govt. of Bihar .

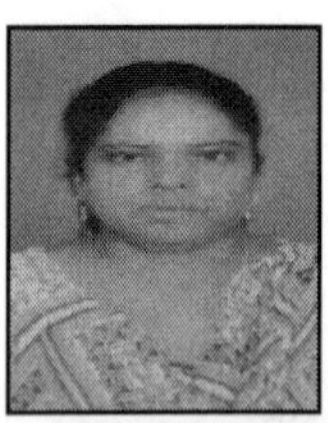

**Dr. Smita Tudu** has done her Ph.D under the supervision of Prof. (Dr.) A. K. Choudhary on Aflatoxin. She has published eight Research papers and she has attended six National Conferences. She has worked as SRF in the Research Project, sponsored by Dept. of Env. Forest and Climate Change, Govt. of Bihar. At present , she is Principal in Upgrade High School, Chatra, Poreyahat, Godda .

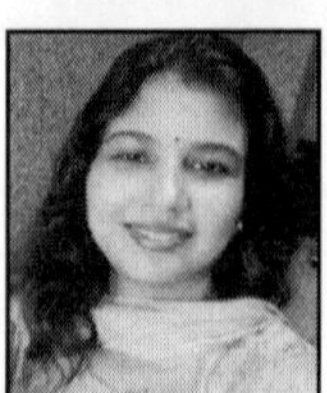

**Dr. (Smt.) Priyanka Kumari** is presently working as Research Officer in the Research Project sponsored by Dept. of Environment, Forest and Climate Change, Govt. of Bihar. She has published approx two dozen research papers in national and international Journals. She has attended 20 National and International Seminars. She has also procured Accession Number (through Gene Bank, Maryland, DNA Data Bank Japan and EMBL, Europe) of nine AFLR gene sequences.

# AFLATOXIN IN CATTLE FEED, MILK AND POSSIBLE CONTROL

A. K. Choudhary
Smita Tudu
Priyanka Kumari

2026

Daya Publishing House®
*A Division of*
Astral International Pvt. Ltd.
New Delhi – 110 002

ISBN: 978-93-5919-269-7



*Published by* : **Daya Publishing House®**
*A Division of*
**Astral International Pvt. Ltd.**
– ISO 9001:2015 Certified Company –
4736/23, Ansari Road, Darya Ganj
New Delhi-110 002
Ph. 011-43549197, 8130496929
E-mail: info@astralint.com
Website: www.astralint.com

*Printed at* : **Replika Press Pvt. Ltd.**

# Preface

Aflatoxins are the secondary metabolities produced mostly by the fungus (Aspergillus species Link ex Fries) and contaminate cattle feed and milk, posing significant health risk to animal and human health. The presence of aflatoxin in food and feed chain has become a growing concern globally, with far reaching implications for dairy industry. The transfer of aflatoxins from contaminated cattle feed to milk is a critical issue that effects not only the dairy industry but also human health and food safety.

The book aims to provide in depth examination of aflatoxin $B_1$ (a potent carcinogen) from cattle feed and milk, its causes, exploring the mechanism of contamination, the factors influencing aflatoxin carry over and the possible control measures. By understanding the complexities of aflatoxin transfer and implementing effective control measures, feed manufactures, dairy farmers and regulatory agencies can work together to minimize the risk associated with aflatoxin contamination and can ensure the safety and quality of milk and dairy products.

Our goal is to equip the professionals, researchers, farmers, dairy technologists and industrialists with the knowledge and update information needed to resolve the challenges posed by aflatoxins and to promote a safer and sustainable cattle feed and dairy industries.

A. K. Choudhary

Smita Tudu

Priyanka Kumari

# Contents

CHAPTER 1

# Introduction

Mycotoxins are secondary metabolites produced by some toxigenic fungi on various food and feed commodities as contaminants. Some of the mycotoxigenic fungi can colonize and penetrate the agricultural crops during any stage of preharvest, harvest, postharvest, processing, as well as storage systems (Bhat *et al.*, 2010). Mycotoxigenic fungi synthesize mycotoxins when the biological, chemical, and physiological and ecological conditions remain conducive. However, this might get sometimes influenced by some geographical, climatological and biological factors such as temperature, types of substrate, moisture content, relative humidity, water activity (aw), co-occurrence of other fungi (taking into account of their synergistic and antagonistic interactions), physical damage inflicted by insects, use of fungicides and storage conditions. There are many other factors which may also influence mycotoxin production such as poor harvesting practices, improper processing, packaging, drying techniques and transport activities.

Climate changes have marked influence on mycotoxin contamination of foods and feedstuffs. As a result of alterations in the environmental and climatic conditions, different fungal species can find opportunity of invasion in food and feedstuff. *Aspergillus, Penicillium, Alternaria* and *Fusarium* species are the principal mycotoxin producers. *Penicillium* and *Aspergillus* species are capable of growing at higher temperature and lower water availability than *Fusarium* and *Alternaria*. Species of *Aspergillus* are ubiquitous and can infest and contaminate a wide range of substrates (cereals, oilseeds, palm kernels, cocoa, vegetables, dryfruits, spices and coffee beans) in addition to air, soil (Kozakiewicz, 1996; Bilgrami and Choudhary, 1996). Depending on the chemical structure and biological origin, mycotoxins can be classified into 4 categories (polyketoacids, terpenes, cyclopeptides, and nitrogenous metabolites). Of the naturally occurring mycotoxins, there are five groups of toxins that are of the greatest concern. These are aflatoxins, ochratoxins, zearalenone, deoxynivalenol and fumonisins (Bianchini & Bullerman, 2014).

The sorry state of affair is, about 25% of the global crop harvests are contaminated with mycotoxins annually which take their toll as huge agricultural and industrial losses measuring into billions of dollars (Marin *et al.*, 2013; Eskola *et al.*, 2019). Among the various mycotoxins, aflatoxins (AFs) are considered as most potent hepatotoxic in livestock and human as well, thereby, creating an extra burden to agriculture sector and even causing significant economic setbacks (Mitchell *et al.*, 2016; Ostry *et al.*, 2017).

Among the various groups of naturally occurring mycotoxins, aflatoxin, produced by different species of *Aspergillus*, especially *A. flavus* Link ex Fries, *A. parasiticus* Speare and *A. nominus* Kurtzman is a secondary metabolite which can enter into the food chain at any stage of crop development. They have been found to contaminate several food commodities including cereals, peanuts, dry fruits, spices and vegetables. Being highly toxic, carcinogenic, mutagenic, teratogenic and immunosuppressive in nature, aflatoxins have been reported as the causal agents in cases of various health complications like Turkey X- disease, Indian Childhood Cirrhosis (ICC), liver cancer, stunted growth etc.

Aflatoxin was discovered in 1960 while investigating a case of mass deaths of Turkey birds in England due to liver disease. Chemically, it is a coumarin nucleus linked to bifuran, either with a pentanone ($AFB_1$) or with the dihydro derivative $AFB_2$) or six-membered lactone ($AFG_1$) and its corresponding derivative ($AFG_2$) (Papp *et al.*, 2002). These four compounds ($B_1$, $B_2$, $G_1$ and $G_2$) are categorized on the basis of the colour of fluorescence (B = blue; G = green) produced by them under long-wave ultraviolet light, when illuminated by their radiations as well as their Rf values. There are six important aflatoxins associated with the group including $B_1$, $B_2$, $G_1$, $G_2$, $M_1$, and $M_2$ where the last two are the metabolic products of the B group of aflatoxins. Studies indicated that the age of animals have also an influence on $AFB_1$ susceptibility. As research indicated that the males are more susceptible than females and young animals of all species are more susceptible than mature animals with regards to the effects of aflatoxins (Mitchell *et al.*, 2016; Krska *et al.*, 2008). Most common of the symptoms of aflatoxicoses on animals include feed refusal, reduced growth rate, decreased feed efficiency, weight loss and diarrhoea. However, bruises and subcutaneous haemorrhage along with anemia are in fact indicative symptoms of aflatoxicoses. The long term effect of aflatoxin inflicted disease may also include impair reproductive efficiency, few or abnormal estrous cycles (too short and too long) and repeated abortions in milching livestock. Not out of place to mention that the symptoms can include impaired immune system response, increased susceptibility to diseases, and prolapsed rectum (Mitcell *et al.*, 2016). Aflatoxin after ingestion is metabolized by cytochrome $P_{450}$ group of enzymes in the liver, where it is converted into aflatoxin 8, 9 epoxide, which in turn forms Guanine moiety after intercalating into DNA. This intercalating of epoxide causes G to T transversion at codon 249 in $P^{53}$ gene in liver, which may lead to hepatic carcinoma.

Contamination of aflatoxin can occur preharvest, harvest, post harvest and storage phases of food and feed grains. Some predisposing factors are essential for preharvest infection *A. flavus* and aflatoxin synthesis. Those factors include availability of toxigenic moulds, susceptible host genotype and conducive climatological factors. In field crop, host-fungus-environmental interactions are the critical factors in determining *A. flavus* infection. In addition, insect damage, drought stress and cultural practices also play significant role in aflatoxin contamination. Once aflatoxin gains foot right in the field conditions, they continue to generate during post harvest and storage conditions. Various factors like high temperature, relative humidity, moisture, substrate, pH and inhabiting microbes influence the synthesis of aflatoxin at various stages of crops (Choudhary, 1992; Sinha and Choudhary, 1993; Bilgrami and Choudhary, 1997; Cassel *et al.*, 2012; Biahchini and Bullerman, 2014).

In the increasing population growth, the safety of food and feed is a matter of major concern. Maize grains are one of the major ingredients of cattle feed. In the finished animal feed the contaminated maize ingredients could cause contamination to the entire feed lot. The consumption of aflatoxin contaminated feed by cattle may cause liver toxicity, physiological alteration, decreased resistance to diseases and also reduced milk production (Sinha and Bhatnagar, 1997; Magan and Olsen, 2004).

Mammals that ingest aflatoxin $B_1$ contaminated diets excrete aflatoxin $M_1$ into milk (also called milk toxins). Aflatoxin $M_1$ ($AFM_1$) is the hydroxylated derivative of aflatoxin $B_1$ and it is found in milk and subsequently in various dairy products when lactating cattle are fed with aflatoxin contaminated feed/ feedstuffs. Several reports have confirmed that aflatoxin $M_1$ is directly correlated to the dietary intake of aflatoxin $B_1$ in cattle feed (Prandini *et al.*, 2007; Mozafari *et al.*, 2017). Milk is supposed to be a complete food and thereby, it is being prescribed to infants, children and old aged people (Bahrami *et al.*, 2016; Costamagna *et al.*, 2019). Those people (infants and old aged people) have comparatively low immunity and therefore, they become more susceptible to the adverse effects of aflatoxin $M_1$. Aflatoxin $M_1$ is genotoxic and it has been categorised as class 2B human carcinogen (IARC 2002). Considering the significance of aflatoxin $M_1$ and its health implications, several countries have imposed stringent law and regulations. European Commission (EU) has set a maximum limit of 0.05 µg/ kg and 20 µg/kg for aflatoxin $B_1$ and total aflatoxins (aflatoxin $B_1$, $B_2$, $G_1$ and $G_2$), respectively (Berg, 2003). Increasing the levels of protein and vitamins A, D, E, K and B in feed help in the efforts to counter the damage, as the toxin binds to vitamins and affects protein synthesis. Better practices adopted for production and storage of feed along with farm management strategies are essential to reduce the risk of secondary infections, where much immediate attention and treatment are needed (Gonzalez *et al.*, 2004).

Mycotoxins particularly aflatoxins could be referred as *enemies under disguise* as they cause numerous undiagnosed health issues and toxicity related illness in farmed livestock globally. However, among the cattle breeders and farmers in general, there is ignorance about the severity of mycotoxin infestation and its uptake. The aflatoxin in feed samples undergoes detoxification in liver and here it gets hydroxylated and secreted into milk (as $AFM_1$). This process of conversion of $AFB_1$ taken by animals into $AFM_1$ present in milk is referred to as-"Carryover". This adds to the gravity of situation as infants all over the world are fed on milk and milk derived baby feed.

$AFM_1$ is mild heat resistant and mild acidic, which is used in the production of milk products (Yoghurt, Cheese, Cream and Butter). Therefore, if milk is contaminated there is the great possibility of $AFM_1$ appearance in dairy products (Colak, 2007; Oruc *et al.*, 2006; Kos *et al.*, 2014). In an investigation, Siddappa *et al.* (2012) investigated the level of aflatoxin $M_1$ in raw, pasteurized, UHT milk samples and found that 48.8% of raw, 42.8% of pasteurized and 64.4% of UHT milk samples contained $AFM_1$ exceeding the EU maximum permissible limits. The pattern of distribution of $AFM_1$ in whey, curd and cheese made from milk (naturally contaminated with $AFM_1$) showed that in comparison with milk, the levels of toxin increased in curd and cheese by 3 and 4.5 folds, respectively, while it decreased in whey by approx 40% (Manetta *et al.*, 2009). It has been reported that $AFM_1$ has high affinity for protein fraction of milk (casein) and thereby, its concentration was higher in cheese compared to milk from where it was derived (Kamkar *et al.*, 2008; Prandini *et al.*, 2009; Ismail *et al.*, 2017).

The rate of carryover from $AFB_1$ to $AFM_1$ in milk in animal is the result of metabolism in the liver and excretion of $AFM_1$ in blood and milk. The rate of this carryover from feed to milk exhibits a wide range of variations. Many investigations suggested that the occurrence of carryover percentage was associated with the milk yields. High percentage has been reported with very high yielding breeds. Cows with the production higher than 28.5l/day showed comparatively high rate of carryover than those cows with lower production of milk (Costamagna *et al.*, 2019). The carryover rate varies from 1 and 3% as per the reports of European Food Safety Authority (EFSA, 2001). In high-producing dairy cows (approx 40l $day^{-1}$ of milk) the rate may reach upto 6%. (Michlig *et al.*, 2016), suggesting that milk production was the main factor affecting the carryover rate. In another reports, $AFB_1$ after being ingested by the livestocks gets transformed into $AFM_1$ in milk, however, carryover rate varied from 0.3 to 6% (Ayar *et al.*, 2007). Aflatoxin $M_1$ contamination in buffalo milk has earlier also been reported in India (Yadgiri and Tulpuley, 1974). Out of 50 milk samples analyzed, 27 samples showed $AFM_1$ in amounts ranging from traces to 4.8µg/l. The toxin level in milk generally remain low as its level in milk is influenced by the molecular weight of the toxin, lipophilicity, pH gradient between the blood plasma and milk and also on animal health status (Kalac, 2011; Algeri *et al.*, 2015). $AFM_1$ may also cross the placental barrier from the pregnant mother animal and thus contaminating the foetus by exposing the newborn to aflatoxin risk whereas human exposure to $AFM_1$ occurs primarily through the milk and milk products from animals that have consumed contaminated feed (Reddy *et al.*, 2007). Taking into account of all these relevant considerations, the predicted rate of $AFB_1$ to $AFM_1$ carry over from feedstuff into milk is approximately 0.3 to 6.0 % (Heshmati & Melani, 2010). The extent of $AFB_1$ conversion into $M_1$ varies greatly and ranges from 0.3 to 6.2% (Var & Kabak, 2009; Ismail *et al.*, 2015). Elevated concentration of $AFB_1$ in feed results in elevated levels of $AFM_1$ in milk and milk products (Klerx *et al.*, 2016). Several factors have been reported to influence the biotransformation of $AFB_1$ to $AFM_1$, those include types of breed, health of the cattle, type of diet (feed types), milk production, rate of ingestion and digestion, metabolism (milk yield, lactation stage) and other factors such as weather and/ or geographical location of dairy farms (Masoero *et al.*, 2007; Duarte *et al.*, 2013). The rate of carryover of $AFB_1$ to $M_1$ also varies among breeds, days and from one milking session to another in addition to physiological factors such as diet and health status of animals especially the status of the liver and its enzymatic activities (Langat *et al.*, 2016).

Mycotoxins in turn have hampered international trade and commerce, wastage of food and feed, and have been the lead factors behind the diversion of huge resources toward's research. The need of the hour is to strict enforcement of regulations to control $AFB_1$ contamination of feed/ food items and applications to alleviate periodical occurrence of mycotoxin problems (Stoev, 2013; Mitchell *et al.*, 2016). However, in an agricultural setup and societal composure like Bihar state of India such regulation should be supported with Government controlled reform and storage management programmes for small and marginal farmers and dairy entrepreneurs.

In Bihar, high population density, floods during the harvesting of maize (major ingredients of cattle feeds), poor harvesting and storage facilities and excessive moistening of the grains adds to the gravity of the problem. Here we have high chances of mould infestation and $AFB_1$ contamination and hence, high incidence of $AFM_1$ occurrence in milk and in milk products cannot be ruled out. Owing to this fact this study was designed with the following objectives.

In the present investigation the survey of cattle feed, milk and milk products of Bhagalpur division was carried out to monitor the level of aflatoxin. The aim of the work was also to study the transfer of $AFB_1$ from feed to milk. Different control strategies were employed to minimize the levels of $AFM_1$ in milk. With those objectives in mind, the research work was carried out with following plan of work:-

(i) Samples of cattle feed, milk and milk products were collected from different areas of Bhagalpur division.

(ii) Analysis of collected samples was done for qualitative and quantitative estimations of aflatoxins.

(iii) Carryover of aflatoxin from cattle feed to milk was evaluated.

(iv) Influence of different variables (seasons, age, individuals) in the carryover rate of aflatoxin was monitored.

(v) Aflatoxin levels were also observed in different components of milk.

(vi) Different control strategies were finally developed to minimize aflatoxin contamination in milk.

CHAPTER 2

# Review of Literature

Mycotoxins have received considerable attention during the past few decades. The term Mycotoxin is amalagamation of Greek word "mykes" and latin word "toxicum" meaning fungus and poison, respectively. The term Mycotoxin is thus now used to designate a group of secondary metabolites produced by certain strains of fungal species that cause illness or death when consumed through natural routes by animals or human beings. Many crops and cereals are susceptible to fungal attack under field or storage conditions. The levels of Mycotoxin contamination in food and feed vary from year to year, depending upon the nature of the host, availability of toxigenic strains and adverse climatic conditions favouring to the fungal invasion and growth. Many of the mycotoxins came into light only when they caused a variety of acute or subacute health problems in animals/ human beings with many of the target organs or systems viz. hepatotoxic, nephrotoxic, neurotoxic, cytotoxic, alimentary tract toxins or esterogenic toxins. Our modern farming, storage and processing practices are aimed to reduce the level of contamination in agriculture and food with the focus to reduce the levels of exposure. Many of the mycotoxins are potent animal carcinogens and have been classified either as human carcinogens or potential carcinogens (IARC, 1993).

However, mycotoxins are toxic, chemically diverse secondary metabolites produced by a wide range of moulds. More than 100 saprophytic moulds have been reported to infest the agricultural crops and elaborate different types of mycotoxins. Mycotoxins are mainly produced by different species of genera viz. *Aspergillus, Penicillium, Alternaria* and *Fusarium*. Infection by moulds and mycotoxin elaboration can take place in the field, during harvesting and/ or during transportation or storage (Martins *et al.*, 2007). Fungal species can be broadly divided into two groups i.e. field fungi and storage fungi. Fungi invading standing crops are referred to as field fungi while those which infest grains in the storage are storage fungi. It is established now that a large number of storage fungi (responsible for post-harvest mycotoxin elaboration) can get associated with the food grains from the fields (pre-harvest stage). Fungi which are found associated with standing crops may not have the potential to infect and grow in the fields owing to the fact that the moulds have fairly better chance of growing in godowns/ warehouses under storage than in fields. However, there are certain moulds which are capable of invading the receptive parts of the plants of the susceptible varieties of crops with parasitic attributes and can successfully grow under field conditions. Temperature, moisture, oxygen, substrate reaction, inoculum concentration, microbial interaction, mechanical damage and insect infection are few important factors that influence the mycotoxin production. Spores of the toxigenic fungi are found ubiquitously in the surrounding of the field crops in soil, water and air and once they find favourable conditions, they can germinate, grow and produce toxins in any part of the crop/ fodder plants. The main sources of mycotoxins in the animal and human food chains are through contaminated agricultural products. Toxigenic fungi can grow and produce mycotoxin on growing crops, seed leaves, stems, fruits, plants and feed. The contamination of mycotoxins can take place before, during and following harvest including during transportations, transit and storage. Apart from agricultural products, animal products may contain mycotoxins resulting from the direct contamination by toxigenic fungi or through the consumption of contaminated feed resulting in secondary mycotoxicoses.

The carry-over of toxin (aflatoxin) into animal products especially milk is a cause of concern, however, the amounts of toxic residues (milk toxins) remain several times lower compared to the feed. In most of the countries of the world milk is a part of nearly all diets. There is a possibility that the toxins may be consumed directly through milk and/ or through dairy products (Betina, 1989). Moreover, certain moulds being used in cheese and food fermentation are also reported to produce mycotoxins (Le Bars, 1979; Pitt *et al.*, 1986; Engel and Teuber, 1989). Other than in natural products, mycotoxigenic fungi are also found in work environments as air-born dust particles or even misused as possible warfare agents and thereby, can result in mycoses.

Mycotoxins induce adverse health effects in both farm and laboratory animals and humans (Malloy and Marr, 1997) depending on dosage or host species susceptibility. They can induce acute or chronic toxicity. Mycotoxins cause different effects in different organs and may ultimately result in death of animals and human beings. Regular monitoring of the presence of mycotoxins is therefore needed. Scientists do not yet know how many mycotoxins may exist even though more than 250 have been detected so far. They represent diverse types of chemicals. For many of those mycotoxnis, their toxicological characteristics have not been fully determined.

## History of Mycotoxins

Fungal poisoning has been recognized since dawn the civilization. Historical reports indicate that the illness caused by fungi had been occurring before the age of ancient Greco-Romans. However, until the end of the nineteenth century, only few scientific observations were made. It was found that consumption of bread made from grain contaminated by *Fusarium* resulted dizziness and headaches in man (Woronin, 1891). During 1850, the intoxication of cattle due to forage poisoning was attributed to the consumption of mould infested feed.

Many mycotoxins and mycotoxigenic fungi of economic consequences were later discovered because they were associated with mycotoxicoses affecting humans (ergotism, liver cancer, yellow rice disease, alimentary toxic aleukia (ATA), Balkan endemic nephropathy (BEN) and red mould toxicoses or animals (Turkey X-disease from aflatoxins, procine nephrapathy from ochratoxin A, vulvo vaginitis in pigs from zearalenone, Equine linkoencephalomalacia (ELEM) and porcine pulmonary edema (PPE) from fumonisins). The examples are ATA, ergotism, starchbotryotoxicosis, and aflatoxicosis.

According to Goldblatt (1972), ingestion of rye infested with *Claviceps purpurea*, induced ergotism was probably the first mycotoxicosis recorded in history. It was suspected to be the cause of periodic outbreaks of "St Anthony's Fire" or St. Vitu's dance that killed several thousand people in Europe. Similar outbreaks also occurred in the 1930's in England and Russia. This disease is caused by different species of *Claviceps purpurea* and *C. paspali*. These fungi grow in the ovaries of grains especially rye and other cereals and produced dark brownish fruiting bodies, sclerotia (also called ergots). These ergots were difficult to be separated from normal grains at the milling and thereby, get dispersed in flour made from those grains. Now it is confirmed that these sclerotia (ergots) containing ergot alkaloids representing acidamide derivatives of D-lysergic acid i.e. ergotamine and alkaloids of ergotoxin group (ergocorine, ergocryptin and ergocristine) which are toxic secondary metabolites of the fungi, *Claviceps*. There are also report of epidemics of ergotism from France (Gabbai *et al.*, 1951), Ethiopia (King, 1970; Dameke *et al.*, 1979) and India (Krishnamachari and Bhat, 1976). Ergotism causes constriction in blood vessels leading to the burning sensation in hands and feet. In extreme cases cell death (necrosis), gangrene and hallucinations may occur resulting into the death.

Another reported serious mycotoxicosis epidemic in human was Alimentary Toxic Aleukia. This disease prevailed in Russia from last century to the end the Second World War. Due to the outbreaks, special organizations were deputed in the then USSR to study the cause of mycotoxicoses (Bilai, 1953; Sarkisov, 1954; Sperivtseva, 1960). However, in general, the effects of mycotoxins were largely ignored in the west and thereby, mycotoxicoses in general were recognized as "The neglected disease". ATA is very unpleasant disease of human beings, disease syndrome included fever, bleeding from skin, nose, throat, gums, necrosis and suppression of immune system. Death due to ATA resulted thousands of population in USSR, especially in the Orenburg district (around the Caspian sea) from 1942-1998 (during world war-II). Later it was recognized that the death was due to consumption of over-wintered millet and buckwheat infested with *Fusarium poe* and *F. sporotrichioides* (*F. trincintum*). Toxins responsible for ATA was later evidenced as trichothecenes. T-2 toxins are also responsible for a variety of diseases both in man and domestic animals. ATA epidemics are also reported from Europe, Japan, Russia and United States (Ueno, 1980). T-2 toxins have also been correlated to be involved in the high incidence of oesophageal cancer in the Republic of Transkie (South Africa) (Marases *et al.*, 1979). Hay infected with *Stachybotrys alterans* when consumed cause diseases primarily in horses and cattle but it also effects human beings. Some of the common symptoms of the disease include dermatitis, buccal inflammation and pain with burning sensation in mouth (Drobotka, 1974). The disease results from a series of trichothecenes toxins designated as satratoxins C, D, F, G and H.

Other mycotoxins which seriously affected the human populations include acute cardiac beriberi in Japan (Uraguchi, 1971) caused by Citreoviridin, the mycotoxin being produced by *Penicillium citreoviride.* Balkan Nephropathy, a fatal renal disease though endemic has been reported from Bulgaria, Romania and Yugoslavia (Barnes, 1967). In fact the landmark year in the history of mycotoxicology is 1960 when over 100,000 young turkeys died in England within short period while consuming contaminated peanut meal imported from Brazil. Later, the disease was called "Turkey-x-Disease" (Blount, 1961). At the same time high incidences of liver disease also occurred in ducklings in Kenya and hatchery reared trout in United States. Subsequent studies revealed that the real etiological agent was the secondary metabolite of the storage moulds *Aspergillus flavus* Link ex Fries (Sargeant *et al.*, 1961). The toxin was named, aflatoxin, according to an abbreviation of *Aspergillus flavus* and toxin. Intensive researches on aflatoxins formed the origin of the modern-day science of mycotoxins and mycotoxicology. However, retrospective studies during 1980's on the Turkey "X" Disease revealed the fact that aflatoxin alone could not induce all symptoms occurring in the turkeys, especially neurotoxic effects. Aflatoxins in association of cyclopiazoic acid (CPA) could explain the symptoms in Turkey 'X' Disease (Cole, 1986). However, possibilities of the co-production of cyclopiozonic acid (CPA) with aflatoxin and their involvement in natural outbreaks of aflatoxicoses cannot be ruled out. (Cole, 1986; Gqualeni *et al.*, 1996). The toxic effects of CPA to induce diseases in animals or humans have also been reported earlier (Harrison, 1971; Rao and Husain 1985).

## Mycotoxigenic Fungi

Till date more than four hundred mycotoxins are known to be produced by different fungi (Jones *et al.*, 1994). However, merely the presence of a fungus does not reflect that a specific toxin or secondary metabolite is present or produced on the foodstuffs. A fungus may co-produce several different mycotoxins. Biosynthesis of secondary metabolites depends on several factors including the nature of the species and strains of moulds. Even the strain of a single species may vary with respect to the quality of toxin produced.

The growth and activity of fungi are greatly influenced by the availability of nutrients pH, radiation, temperature and water activity interactions. Moreover, biological and chemical agents such as acid treatment, pH change due to lactic acid fermentation may also influence the development of moulds in mycotoxin bioynthesis.

Today more than 18,000 fungal secondary metabolites have been reported, however, only a restricted number has received the scientific interest from the 1960's and onwards (Cole and Cox, 1981). The most studied are regulated mycotoxins i.e., aflatoxins (AFs), critinin, trichiothecenes such as deoxynivalenol (DON), patulin, ochratoxin A (OTA), fumonisins (FBs) and zearalenone (ZEA) and some major toxins of endophytic fungi (ergot toxins and ergotamine).

**Table 1:** Some important mycotoxigenic fungi and mycotoxicoses

| **Mycotoxincoses / Causative mycotoxins** | **Main toxigenic fungi** | **Animal species** | **Main susceptible crops** |
|---|---|---|---|
| Aflatoxicoses, Aflatoxin - $B_1$, $B_2$, $G_1$, $G_2$ | *Aspergillus flavus*<br>*A. parasiticus*<br>*A. homius* | poultry, swine, cattle | corn, small grains, peanuts, cottonseeds, cassava, copra, nut crops, cattle feeds. |
| Ergotism<br>Ergotamine, ergotoxin and ergometrine alkaloids | *Claviceps purpurea* | poultry, cattle, sheep, swine | rye, wheat, barley, rice, millet, sorghum, triticale. |
| Zearalenone toxicoses | *Fusarium spp.* | Swine, rat cattle | corn, wheat, barley, sorghum, oats |
| Trichothecenes toxicoses T-2 toxin, diacetoxyscirpelnol, vomitoxin and others | *Fusarium spp.* | swine, cattle, poultry | corn, wheat, barley, oats, millet, rye, mixed feeds. |
| Leucoencephalomalacia | *Fusarium moniliforme* | Horse | Corn |
| Ochratoxicoses<br>Ochratoxin A, B | *Aspergillus ochraceus* | swine, poultry | corn, oats, barley, bean, peanuts, mixed feeds. |
| Citrinin toxicoses | *Penicillium spp.* | swine, poultry | wheat, rye, oats, barley |
| Cyclopiazonic acid | *Aspergillus flavus*<br>*A. orazae*<br>*Penicillium camemberti*<br>*P. candidum*<br>*P. griseofulvum*<br>*P. patulum*<br>*P. viridicatum*<br>*P. puberulum*<br>*P. crustosum* | Diverse animals, cattles | corn, peanuts, soil, grain, pepper, cacao, pistachios, cheese, meat, peanuts, cured ham, fermented sausage, raw ham |

| | | | |
|---|---|---|---|
| Tenuazonic acid (TA),<br>Alternariol (AOH),<br>Alternariol methyl ether (AME)<br>Altenuene (ALT)<br>Altertoxin – I (ATX-I) | *Alternaria spp.* | Dog, cat and chicken | Wheat, Sorghum |

## Effect of Mycotoxins

Mycotoxins are the secondary metabolites produced by fungus which are chemically unrelated and have deleterious effect on other living organisms including human to the extent that might lead to death and are harmful even to green plants. These chemical compounds are produced by certain toxigenic moulds during their development on food and feed materials. Mycotoxicoses is defined as a series of toxicity related symptoms produced by the consumption of Mycotoxin containing food and feed.

Apart from agricultural products, animal products may contain mycotoxins resulting from the direct contamination by toxigenic fungi or the consumption of contaminated fed by animals resulting in secondary mycotoxicoses. Figure 1 clearly describes primary or secondary mycotoxicoses.

Today more than 350 mycotoxins have been characterized and the studies suggest that major research have been carried on aflatoxin and tricothecenes along with some other important mycotoxins viz. Ochratoxins, putulin, sterigmatocystin, citrinin, cyclopiazonic acid and zearalenone.

**Table 2:** Important mycotoxins and their target organs.

| | | |
|---|---|---|
| (A) | Hepatotoxins | Aflatoxins<br>Sporidesmin<br>Luteoskyrin<br>Cyclochlorotine<br>Rubratoxins<br>Sterigmatocystin |
| (B) | Nephrotoxins | Ochratoxins<br>Citrinin |
| (C) | Neurotoxins | Penitrem<br>Patulin<br>Citreoviridins<br>Miscellaneous neurotoxins<br>Ergots |

| | | |
|---|---|---|
| (D) | Cytotoxins (alimentary tract toxins) | Trichothecenes<br>T-2 toxins<br>Diacetoxyscirpenol<br>Neosolaniol<br>Nivalenol<br>Deoxynivalenol (DON, Vomitoxin)<br>HT-2 toxin |
| (E) | Esterogenic mycotoxins | F-2 toxins (Zearalenone) |

## Potential Health Implications of Mycotoxins

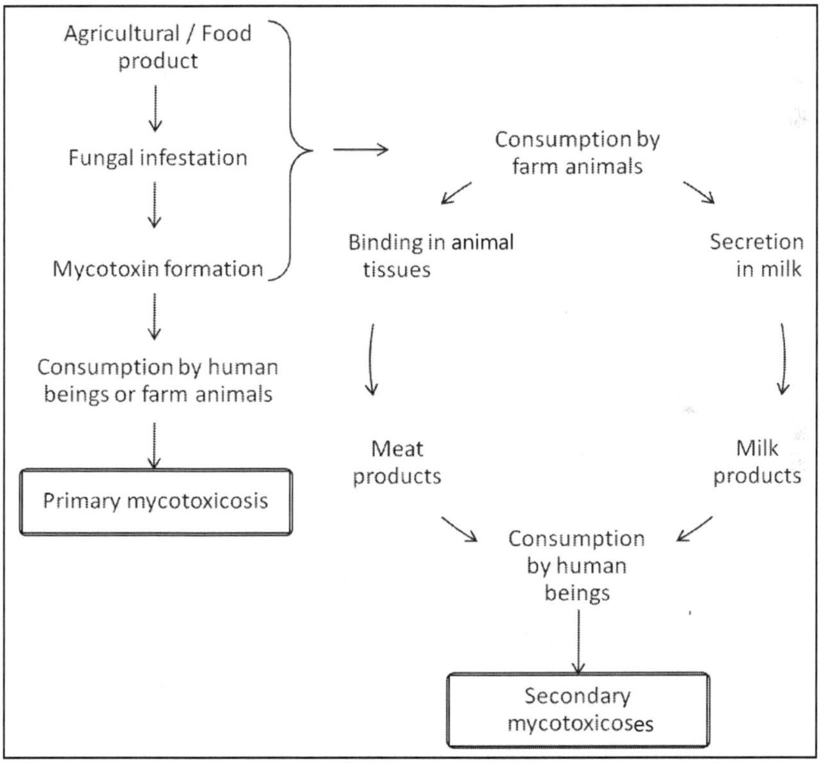


**Fig. 1:** Primary and secondary mycotoxicoses.

**Table 3:** Possible involvement of mycotoxins in some human diseases

| Implicated mycotoxins | Mycotoxicosis |
|---|---|
| Aflatoxin | Aflatoxicoses (acute)<br>Hepatocarcinogenesis<br>Indian Childhood cirrhosis<br>Reye's syndrome<br>Encephalopathy and fatty degeneration of the viscera |
| Amatoxin, agaritine amanitins, Phallotoxins etc. | Kwashiorkar, Mushroom poisoning |
| Citreoviridin | Cardiac beriberi |
| Cyclopiazonic acid | Kodua poinsoning |
| Ergot alkaloids | Ergotism |
| Gliotoxin | Lung disease |
| Moniliformin | Onyalai disease, Oesophageal cancer |
| Ochratoxin | Balkan nephropathy, renal tumors |
| Trichothecenes DAS, HT-2, FUS-X | Alimentary toxic aleukia<br>Akakabi-byo disease<br>Kaschin-Bech disease |
| *F. oxysporum metabolites* | Stachybotryotoxicosis |
| *Stachy botrys alternans metabolites* | Esophageal cancer |
| Fusarium metabolites | Red mould disease |
| DON, DAS, T-2 | Yellow rain |
| Tenuazonic acid | Onyalai disease |
| Zearalenone | Cervical cancer, follicular growth disorder, onset of puberty, Premature thelarche |

## Effect of Mycotoxins on Plant Systems

Mycotoxins can also cause a series of physiological and biochemical distress/ disorders in higher plants, ferns and also in microbes (algae, fungi and bacteria) (Reiss, 1978; Chohan, 1983; Bilgrami and Sinha, 1985).

## Effect on Higher Plants

Aflatoxins can inhibit plant growth through inhibition of seed germination and the formation of seedlings. Subsequent inhibition in seed germination of *Lipidium sativum* was reported by Schoental and White (1965). Reiss (1973) observed that lower concentration of aflatoxin (10 ppm) induced chlorophyll deficiency in the same plant, whereas higher concentration completely inhibited seed germination and radical development.

Seed germination of different species of crucifers was not affected by 100 ppm of aflatoxin $B_1$, although the formation of the hypocotyl and radicle was found to be severely affected by the toxin (Crisan, 1973). In Cowpea, seed germination was inhibited both by aflatoxin $B_1$ and by crude aflatoxins (Adekunle and Bassir, 1973). Seed soaking with the filtrate of aflatoxigenic strains of *A. flavus* resulted in the inhibition of seed germination. In case of *Phaseolus oureus*, there was 100% inhibition of seed germination (Sinha and Kumari, 1989). Aflatoxin $B_1$ has been shown to inhibit seed germination of Sorghum (Tripathi, 1973), maize (Jeswal, 1987) and mung (Sinha and Kumari, 1989).

Aflatoxin $B_1$ cause the inhibition of chlorophyll synthesis in the cotyledonary leaves of *Abelmoschus esculentum* (Kang, 1970; Mehan, 1971). The affected plants show symptoms like virescence and albinism due to inhibition of chlorophyll synthesis. Electron microscopic studies of the leaves of maize demonstrated that there was inhibition in grana formation in the chloroplast (Slowatlizky *et al.*, 1969; Jacquet *et al.*, 1971). Chlorophyll formation was also reported to be adversely affected by aflatoxin in developing cotyledonary leaves of Cucumber (*Cucumis sativus*). Chohan (1983) demonstrated that aflatoxin alters Chlorophyll synthesis by inhibiting the synthesis of growth hormone which in turn effect the synthesis of DNA, RNA and Protein.

Aflatoxin $B_1$ suppressed the synthesis of RNA, DNA and Protein in germinating seeds of Maize (Sinha and Kumari, 1989) and mung (Sinha and Kumari, 1989). Aflatoxins at subtoxic concentration causes inhibition in the DNA dependent RNA polymerase activity (Tripathi and Mishra, 1983). Dashek and Liewellyn (1974) reported that aflatoxin $B_1$ interferes with protein synthesis in germinating pollen of *Lillium longiflorum*.

Aflatoxigenic moulds and aflatoxins both adversely affect the nutritive value of several agricultural produce as they have been reported to significantly lower the levels of sugars, proteins, phenols, ascorbic acid and also the caloric value in Maize (Bilgrami *et al.*, 1979, 1981), fleshy fruits (Singh and Sinha, 1982; Sinha and Singh, 1982) and dry fruits (Bilgrami *et al.*, 1983).

Aflatoxin also induces cytological abnormalities such as increase of chromosomal numbers during anaphase and significant inhibition of mitosis in *Vicia faba* (Lilly, 1965). In another observation Reiss (1975) reported mycotoxins to induce severe reduction of mitosis and formation of chromosomal bridges. Moreover, contrasting results were obtained by Bilgrami *et al.* (1986) in *Allium cepa* root tips, where low doses of $AFB_1$ were mitoinhibitory while higher doses were found to be mitopromotive. Another mycotoxins such as T-2 toxins have also been reported to have adverse effect on seed germination and seedling growth of *Vigna radiata* L. (Bilgrami *et al.*, 1991). Rahman (1992) also recorded the effect of zearalenone on the seed germination of maize and mung which had significant effect only above the level of 1 ppm.

In case of barley seedlings it was observed that seed germination was inhibited due to inhibition in - amylase activities. Even Gibberellic acid (growth promoting substance) did not alter the inhibitory induction (Nummi *et al.*, 1975). Borthalice *et al.*,1980 reported that DON (Deoxynivalenol) at the concentration of 6 µg /ml inhibited almost completely the growth of Tomato seedlings. T-2 toxin and several other trichothecenes have been reported to cause electrolyte leakage from tomato leaf discs (Pavlakin et al., 1986). (Cole *et al.*, 1981) have shown T-2 toxin influences inhibition of elongating Wheat coleoptiles.

Chromosomal aberrations and adverse effect on mitotic frequency were observed in *Allium* root tip treatments with fusarial toxins (Reiss, 1975). Recently Packa (1991) has observed reduction in mitotic index and chromosomal abnormalities in cereals (rye/ wheat/ triticales) when the seeds were treated with the solutions of DON and DAS at the concentration of 10µg/ ml. DNA and RNA contents in maize and mung seeds were adversely effected by Zearelenone (Rahman, 1992). Fusarial toxin influences hormonal balance of the host plant. There are the reports that DAS breaks the dormancy of lateral buds in *Vicia faba* (Brian *et al.*, 1961). However, these toxins have deleterious effects on the apical buds.

## Effect on Lower Plants

Cahilol et al. (1978) studied the effect of aflatoxin $B_1$ on germination and protoxemal development of a fern. *Onclea sensibilis* and noted 50% reduction in spore germination at 12.5 µg/ ml aflatoxin concentration; increasing concentration caused reduction in the total number of cells per protonema. Inhibition of the growth of *Chlorella pyrenoidosa* was recorded at 4µg of aflatoxin $B_1$ ml in liquid culture and at 12.5 µg/ disk assay method (Ikawa *et al.*, 1969). Lillihoj et al, (1967a) reported inhibition of the growth of *Aspergillus flavus, A. awamori, Penicillium chrysogenum* and *P. duelauxi* by aflatoxin $B_1$. Aflatoxins also effected fermentation capabilities of yeast strains (Reiss, 1973). Zearalenone reduced the formation of fungal *perthicia* at low concentration, however, it inhibited the growth of *Chlorella pyrenoidosa* and *Bacillus megaterium* (Sullivan and Ikawa, 1972).

## Aflatoxins

Aflatoxins are synthesized in polyketide pathway and are difuranocoumarin derivative produced by strains of *Aspergillus flavus* and *A. parasiticus*. Among different types of aflatoxins produced by *A. flavus* strains, aflatoxin $B_1$ is extremely toxic, mutagenic and carcinogenic (Richard *et al.*, 2003, Ismaiel; 2014). Numerous studies have been conducted to determine the effects of various food additives, preservatives, chemicals and environmental conditions to inhibit growth and aflatoxin production effectively (Chipley *et al.*, 1980, Paranagama *et al.*, 2003, Krishnamurthy *et al.*, 2006, Gnonlonfin *et al.*, 2011, Ismaiel *et al.*, 2011, Pratiwi *et al.*, 2015). Toxigenic *A. flavus* isolates mostly produce either $B_1$, $B_1$ $G_1$ and $B_1$ $G_1$ $B_2$, however, toxigenic *A. parasiticus* strains produce all the four aflatoxins ($B_1$, $B_2$, $G_1$ and $G_2$) (Cotty *et al.* 1994). Aflatoxin $B_1$ is carcinogen and is excreted in milk in the form of aflatoxin $M_1$. Aflatoxins often occur in crop in the field prior to harvest. Post-harvest contamination can occur if crop drying is delayed and also during storage if water exceeds the critical value for mold growth (Bilgrami and Choudhary, 1998).

## Physical and Chemical Properties of Aflatoxins

Aflatoxins in crystalline state remain colourless to pale yellow. They fluoresce under long wave ultraviolet (UV) light. They are soluble in moderately polar solvents viz. chloroform, methanol and dimethyl solfoxide (DMSO) and are insoluble in non polar solvents, which, however, is sparingly soluble in water. Aflatoxins in pure state are stable at high temperature but relatively unstable when exposed to light and UV radiation. Physical and chemical properties of some important aflatoxins and their metabolites are represented in Table- 4, 5. Aflatoxins are highly oxygenated heterocyclic coumarin derivative compounds. Now a days more than two dozen aflatoxins (their derivatives) are known which include $B_1$, $B_2$, $B_{2a}$, $B_3$, $G_1$, $GM_1$, $G_2$, $G_{2a}$, $M_1$, $M_2$, $M_{2a}$, $GM_2$, $P_1$, $R_1$, $R_0$, $RB_1$, $RB_2$, AFL, AFLH, AFLM, methoxy, ethoxy and aceto derivatives. While considering the toxicity different aflatoxins can be graded in descending order as $AFB_1 > AFB_2 > AFG_1 > AFG_2$, respectively.

In the lactating cow, aflatoxin gets hydroxylated. $AFM_1$ and $AFM_2$ are the hydroxylation products of 4$^{th}$ carbon of $AFB_1$ and $AFB_2$ molecules, respectively.

Taking structure into accounts $AFB_1$, $AFB_2$, $AFG_1$, $AFG_2$, $AFM_1$ and $AFM_2$ are some of the most common aflatoxins. The term "B" and "G" refer to the colors blue and green fluorescence of UV light on TLC plates while the number 1 and 2 show the respective minor and major compounds (Bennett, 2003). Aflatoxin $B_1$ ($C_{17}H_{12}O_6$) exhibits string blue fluorescence under high wavelength. On the other hand, aflatoxin $G_1$ ($C_{17}H_{12}O_7$) exhibits a green fluorescence under high wavelength of UV.

The structural identification of $AFM_1$ was for the first time made through thin layer chromatography (TLC) of the extract of milk. Later on (De Jongh *et. al.*, 1964) showed blue-violet fluorescent compound which had lower $R_f$ value than $AFB_1$. The chromatographic results have revealed that during the lactating period, $AFB_1$ get bio-converted to another toxic compound (toxic milk) which was later assigned the name "Aflatoxin M" (Allcroft *et al.*, 1966).

Stereo-chemistry of aflatoxin in the B and G series by chemical degradation were also elucidated. Structurally, these toxins are coumaryl derivatives having fine rings along with a six membered furfuran moiety (ring) and another six membered lactone ring. $M_1$ and $M_2$ which bear a hydroxy group at the junction of the two furan rings. In some aflatoxins, the D-ring ($RB_1$), $RB_2$ or the E-ring $B_3$ are opened. Their molecular formulas as established from elemental analyses and mass spectrometric determinations are: $AFB_1$ – $C_{17}H_{12}O_6$; $AFB_2$ – $C_{17}H_{14}O_6$; $AFG_1$ – $C_{17}H_{12}O_7$; and $AFG_2$ – $C_{17}H_{14}O_7$ Table 4. $AFB_2$ and $AFG_2$ were established as the dihydroxyl derivatives of $AFB_1$ and $AFG_1$, respectively. Whereas, $AFM_1$ is 4-hydroxyl $AFB_1$ and $AFM_2$ is 4-dihydroxyl $AFB_2$ (Eaton and Groopman, 1994).

Aflatoxin $B_1$ and $G_1$ are the most potent toxins among all the toxins. Other aflatoxins seem to be of less importance with respect to their effects. The structural formulae of some major aflatoxins are illustrated in Fig 2. The initial attention on aflatoxin researches were primarily focused on post-harvest mycology, pathology and its toxicological manifestations in animals. However, later on it was evidenced that aflatoxigenic moulds can infect the crops even in the field conditions. In the present decade aflatoxin has become a major problem because of its extensive preharvest contamination of some important cereal crops (Bilgrami and Choudhary, 1998), cotton seed, treenut (Klich, 2007), mustard (Bilgrami *et al.*, 1992), linseed (Ottalico *et al.*, 1998) and sorghum (Divakara *et al.*, 2014).

**Table 4:** Physical and chemical properties of aflatoxins.

| Aflatoxins | Chemical formula | Molecular Weight | Optical density | | Melting point |
|---|---|---|---|---|---|
| $B_1$ | $C_{17}H_{12}O_6$ | 312 | 268 – 269 | 21,800 | 425 |
| $B_2$ | $C_{17}H_{14}O_6$ | 314 | 286 – 289 | 23,400 | 425 |
| $G_1$ | $C_{17}H_{12}O_7$ | 328 | 244 – 246 | 10,000 | 450 |
| $G_2$ | $C_{17}H_{12}O_7$ | 330 | 327 – 240 | 21,000 | 450 |
| $M_1$ | $C_{17}H_{12}O_7$ | 328 | 299 | 19,000 (357nm) | 425 |
| $M_2$ | $C_{17}H_{14}O_7$ | 330 | 293 | – | – |
| $B_2A$ | $C_{17}H_{14}O_7$ | 330 | 240 | 20,000 | – |
| $G_2A$ | $C_{17}H_{14}O_8$ | 346 | 190 | 18,000 | – |

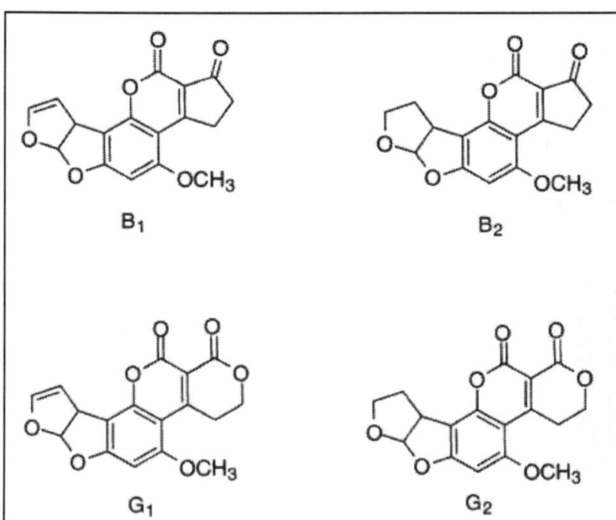

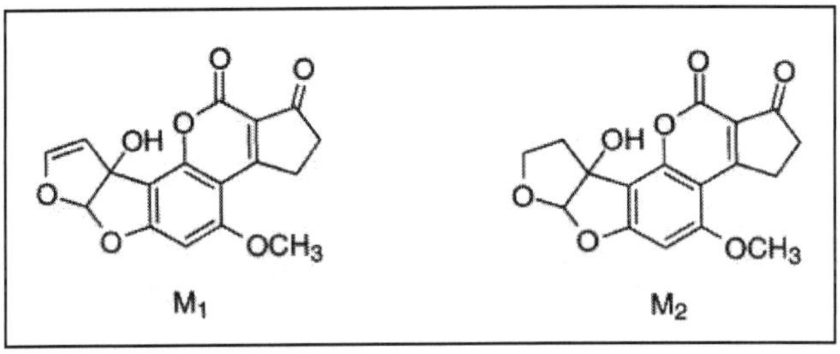


**Fig. 2:** Chemical structure of diffrent affatoxins

**Table 5:** Melting points and ultraviolet absorption of aflatoxins.

| Aflatoxin | Melting point ( C) | Ultra violet absorption | |
|---|---|---|---|
| | | max (nm) | (L–Mol–1cm–1) 103 |
| B1 | 268 – 269 (decomposition) (crystals from $CHCl_3$) | 223 | 25.6 |
| | | 265 | 13.4 |
| | | 262 | 21.8 |
| B2 | 268 – 269 (decomposition) (crystals from $CHCl_3$ – Methanol) | 265 | 11.7 |
| | | 363 | 23.4 |
| G1 | 244 – 246 (decomposition) (crystals from $CHCl_3$ – Methanol) | 243 | 11.5 |
| | | 257 | 9.9 |
| | | 264 | 10.0 |
| | | 362 | 16.0 |
| G2 | 237 – 240 (decomposition) (crystals from ethyl acetate) | 265 | 9.7 |
| | | 363 | 21.0 |
| M1 | 299 (decomposition) (crystals from Methanol) | 226 | 23.1 |
| | | 265 | 11.6 |
| | | 357 | 19.0 |

## Factors Influencing Aflatoxin Synthesis

Like other *Aspergillus* species, *A. flavus* has a worldwide distribution. This probably results from production of numerous airborne conidia, which get dispersed by air movements and also by insects. Among the different climatological factors, relative humidity (RH) is one of the most important variables. Atmospheric composition has a great impact on mould growth, with humidity being the most important variable. *A. flavus* grows better in the water activity between 0.86 and 0.96 (Diener *et al.,* 1987). The optimum temperature for *A. flavus* grows at its optimal potentials at 37 C, however, its growth have been observed at a wide temperature ranging from 12 to 48 C. *A. flavus* is mostly saprophytic, however, it has ability to act as weak parasitic with the increase in temperature. The ability of *A. flavus* to survive in harsh conditions allows it to compete with other organisms on substrates soil or in the standing crops (Bhatnagar *et al.,* 2000).

*A. flavus* can colonize and contaminate grain before harvest or during storage of the host crops. Susceptible crops in field condition get infected with *Aspergillus* when exposed to prolonged high temperature and high humidity or damage from stressful conditions (drought, or in a condition which lowers the barrier to entry). The natural habitat of *Aspergillus* is soil, decaying vegetation, hay and grains undergoing microbiological deterioration and it invade all types of organic substrates whenever conditions are congenial for its growth.

Aflatoxin production by *Aspergillus* reaches its maximum production rate at the fifth day when moulds attain the stationary growth phase. From the sixth to the eight days aflatoxin production diminishes. If optimal conditions of temperature (27.30°C) and relative humidity (85%) are being provided, *Aspergillus flavus* starts synthesizing aflatoxins from 24 hours and produces it upto 12 days, later its rate lowers progressively.

Presence of $CO_2$ and $O_2$ also influence mould growth as well as aflatoxin production. A 20% level of $CO_2$ in the surrounding air depresses aflatoxin production due to marked depression in the mould growth. On the other hand, decrease in the $O_2$ concentration of air to 100%, the growth and aflatoxin production are completely inhibited. Lillehoj (1983) investigated that reduced oxygen or increase carbon dioxide level reduce the fungal activity and toxin production. The maximum production of aflatoxin occurs at pH 5.5. Generally, the preferred carbon sources for aflatoxin production are glucose, sucrose or fructose, however, xylose, ribose and glycerol have also been reported as suitable carbon sources for aflatoxin production. Yeast extract and peptone are good inorganic sources whereas, aspartate, glycine and glutamate are suitable amino acids (organic sources) for aflatoxin production. Mangnese and Zinc are essential for aflatoxin biosynthesis, but a mixture of cadmium and iron depressed mould growth and aflatoxin production.

Several factors affect the growth of *Aspergillus* fungi and the level of aflatoxin contamination in food. Contamination by *Aspergillus* and aflatoxins can occur at any or all stages of the growth and development of crop production starting from preharvest to the storage of the produce (Wilson and Payne, 1994). Various factors such as climatic condition of the region under investigation, crop genotype, soil texture, daily temperature variations, net evaporation and precipitations all influence the mould infection and contamination process by *Aspergillus*. Aflatoxin contamination is also promoted by stress or damage of the crops due to drought prior to harvest, insect activity, timing of harvest and inadequate drying of the crop before storage. Relative humidity, temperature, aeration, drying and storage also influence the growth and aflatoxin biosynthesis in different ways.

## Aflatoxin Effect on Animals

For over forty years, since the beginning with the documentation of Turkey X disease in 1960, the effects of aflatoxins on animal health have been observed in many other species too (Blount, 1961). The liver of animals is the first and common target of aflatoxins. Aflatoxins cause various degrees of hepatotoxicoses. Acute effects include hemorrhagic necrosis of the liver duct proliferation while chronic effects include hepato-cellular carcinoma (HCC). Aflatoxin can induce other adverse affects on animals viz. growth retardation, immune suppression along with enhanced susceptibility towards disease and infections. However, aflatoxin $B_1$ ($AFB_1$) is a highly toxic compound with a lethal dose (LD 50 = 1-50 mg $Kg^{-1}$) for most species, however, its toxicity is critical (LD 50 < 1 mg $Kg^{-1}$) for some highly sensitive species, such as rats, rainbow trout and poultry. Level/ doses of toxic exposure along with the duration of exposure to $AFB_1$ level lead to varied toxic manifestations (Diaz *et al.*, 2011). As an immunomodulator, it retards the resistance to disease and even interferes with vaccine induced immunity in livestock (Diekman and Green, 1992). The overall productivity and health of dairy livestock are severely compromised at levels higher than 100ppb of aflatoxin exposure. It was reported by Guthrie (1979) that dairy animals having upto 120 ppm of aflatoxin exposure exhibit reduced reproductive potentials, while changing to a aflatoxin free diet even enhanced the milk production by 25%. Aflatoxins are immunosuppressive in variety of animals making them more susceptible to infection by various other micro-organisms.

## Effects of Aflatoxin on Human Beings

The effects of aflatoxins on humans, as well as on animals are dependent on dosage and duration of exposure. Prolonged high exposure of aflatoxin results in aflatoxicoses (hepatotoxicity). Early symptoms of hepatoxicity include anorexia, malaise and low-grade fever. Acute high level exposure can progress to potentially lethal hepatitis with vomiting, abdominal pain, Jaundice, fulminant hepatic failure and subsequent death of the patient. One of the recurring public health problems is outbreak of acute aflatoxicoes throughout the world (Bhat et al., 1975; Johnson et al., 1982; Lye, Ghazali *et al.*, 2004). Hepatocellular carcinoma (HCC) as a result of chronic exposure has been well documented, however, generally in association with hepatitis B virus or other risk factors. IARC, 1976 (The International Agency for Research on Cancer) has recognized aflatoxins $B_1$ as carcinogenic for the first time and since then it has been reaffirmed as Class I or Group 1 carcinogens (humans) (IARC, 2002). Chronic exposure and the effects of aflatoxin have been widely studied and it has been suggested to have immunosuppression, retardation of growth and nutritional changes (Phillips *et al.*, 2004). Mycotoxin contamination in food chain is considered as one of the challenging food safety issues throughout the world. Liu and Wu in 2010 have reported that aflatoxins cause 0.025 – 0.15 million cases of hepatic cancer annually. $AFM_1$, although ten times less carcinogenic as compared to $AFB_1$, $B_1$ Group 2B by the International Agency for Research on Cancer (IARC, 2002). European commission (EC) has set a permissible limit of $AFM_1$ in animal milk as 0.05μg/L (EC, 2006). The elevated levels of aflatoxin $M_1$ may also result in hepatocellular carcinoma, immunosuppression as well as teratogenic and mutagenic effects including impairment of kidney and liver (Zheng *et al.*, 2013).

## Biosynthesis of Aflatoxins

Aflatoxins are formed from the precursor, versiconal hemiacetal acetate (benzylated) compound, versiconal hemiacetal acetate is formed from acetate, the units of which are converted into a polyketide. The polyketide is then metabolized to the xanthone versiconal hemiacetal acetate (Bromination at the a-position to the carbonyl group, and conversion into the benzyl ether gave acetal). Intermediate versiconal hemiacetal acetate get converted into versicolorin A or versicolorin B in several steps. Versicolorin A may be converted to sterigmatocystin, while versicolorin B can lead to dihydro-sterigmatocystin. Sterigmatocystin get metabolized to $AFG_1$ or $AFB_1$ which subsequently be transformed to $AFM_1$. Aflatoxins $B_2$ and $G_2$ are formed from dihydrosterigmatocystin and $M_2$ is formed by conversion from $B_2$. Pathways also exist to convert aflatoxin $B_1$ to $B_2$, $M_1$ to $M_2$, and $G_1$ to $G_2$, and vice versa.

## Aflatoxin in Cattle Feed

The occurrence of aflatoxins in feed is a major problem for farmers due to both intoxication (acute and chronic) in animals and subsequently to human. The most common source of aflatoxin contamination of cattle fed is the infestation of potentially toxigenic *Aspergillus flavus*, in agricultural produce like cereals and oil seeds (rice, corn, peanut, cottonseed, millet or sorghum) and some other grains and products which are the principal ingredients of feed formulations. Aflatoxin is the most problematic in diary due to its derivative aflatoxin $M_1$ ($AFM_1$) transferred to milk and its potential health hazard for human especially infants. The studies of contamination of aflatoxins in agricultural commodities like maize, rice, wheat and other crops including oilseeds like peanuts have been reported in many parts of world from various research institutes (Bilgrami and Choudhary, 1998; European Union, 2011; Organuri and Olarewaju, 2013; Hashemi, 2016). The natural occurrence of aflatoxins in various feed material were reported which indicate the contamination of aflatoxins is threat to health (Santini and Ritieni, 2013; Kumar *et al.*, 2016; Sarma *et al.*, 2017; Mushed *et al.*, 2019). Most formulated cattle feed utilizing rice bran as ingredients have been reported to contain aflatoxin. This might be due to the fact that rice bran was contaminated with aflatoxin under natural condition.

Monitoring of aflatoxin $B_1$ in livestock feeds using ELISA and HPLC in Korea was investigated (Han *et al.*, 2005). Smith *et al.* (1994) and Lee *et al.* (2002) have reported that the all four principal aflatoxins $B_1$, $B_2$, $G_1$ and $G_2$ ($AFB_1$, $AFB_2$, $AFG_1$ and $AFG_2$) are potent agents of hepato carcinomas in various animals and human. Ketinagu *et al.*, 2015 investigated assessment of aflatoxin $B_1$ in livestock feed and feed ingredients by high-performance this layer chromatography in Telangana, India. Taking into account of the development in Codex alimentarius, EC has set 20ppb as maximum limit in all feed stuffs for livestocks (cattle, sheep, goat, pigs and poultry). The general standard for all common feed stuffs in 0.05 mg/kg, for dairy animals and 0.01 mg/kg for calves and lambs. The level of aflatoxin in animals are important concern for human health as 1-2% of aflatoxin $B_1$ finds its way into animal milk in the form of aflatoxin $M_1$. Therefore, aflatoxin $B_1$concentration in feed above standards may result in milk containing a higher aflatoxin $M_1$ (Oruce *et al.*, 2007).

In another investigation, Hashemi (2015) observed aflatoxin $B_1$ levels in feedstuffs from dairy cow farms in South of Iran. Aflatoxin $B_1$ contamination and its concentration was determined in 144 dairy farms (cow) and altogether 359 different cow feed samples collected from different parts of Iran were tested. The contamination rate and overall mean level of $AFB_1$ in the samples were 94.8% and 4.12 ± 0.53 µg/kg, respectively. Out of those, 36 samples (10.94%) contained $AFB_1$ level higher than the set limits of 5µg/kg in Iran and EU. The $AFB_1$ level was exceedingly higher than the acceptable limits in Iran for crops such as Corn, Alfalfa hay and Soybean meal etc. The time of sampling unlike the geographical region ($p<0.05$) affected the $AFB_1$ levels in destined feedstuffs for dairy farms.

Ismail et al. (2017) investigated seasonal variation of aflatoxin $B_1$ content in dairy feed of Pakistan. $AFB_1$ level was monitored in three different types of animal feed comprising commercially available animal feed, fresh fodder and leftover bread fed to dairy animals between October 2014 and September 2015. $AFB_1$ was found in all collected samples at the levels over the EU permissible limits (5µg/kg). Mean maximum and mean minimum levels were observed in the winter and summer months, respectively. Study in this regard substantiated the fact that commercial feed and left over breads contained higher $AFB_1$ incidence and hence, there is the need of strict regulatory measures. Higher level of aflatoxin $B_1$ was found to be prevalent in poultry (Bibin Becha, 2013) and other animal feeds (Britzi *et al.*, 2013; Bagheri *et al.*, 2014). $AFB_1$ present in dairy animal feeds is biodegraded in liver and transferred into milk in the form of aflatoxin $M_1$ ($AFM_1$). In Pakistan high levels of aflatoxin contamination has been reported (Chohan *et al.*, 2016; Ullah *et al.*, 2016), however, systematic survey and surveillance of aflatoxin $B_1$ levels in cattle feed samples need to be monitored round the year.

Mohamad and Hermanto (2017) investigated HPLC ultraviolet – photodiode array detection method for aflatoxin $B_1$ in cattle feed supplements in Indonesia. Setlem *et al.* (2016) reported that there was an upsurge of aflatoxin poisoning of cattle feed which made a high concern in East Java province of Indonesia. This was due to a number of upcoming small industries which were producing untreated cattle feed instead of utilizing product quality and sanitation related practices and standards.

Nishimwe *et al.* (2019) evaluated the aflatoxin and Fumonism contamination in feed and feed ingredients along with the risk they posed on animal and human health in Rwanda. They reported that consumption of contaminated feed caused detrimental effects on health and productivity of cattle. For several months if a dairy herd is exposed to contaminated feed (120 µg/kg of aflatoxin) showed severe health problems and a decrease in milk production up to 28%. Lactating mammals metabolites and excrete 6% of $AFB_1$ into milk as $AFM_1$ (Britzi *et al.*, 2013;

Churchill, 2017). Aflatoxin $M_1$ ($AFM_1$) is a metabolite of aflatoxin $B_1$ ($AFB_1$) that is excreted in urine, bile, faeces and milk after dietary exposure of dairy cattle contaminated feed (Algari *et al.*, 2016). Minagri (2018) evidenced the Government efforts to increase dietary, diversity and human nutrition in the countryside of Kenya through Girinka programme (which pertains to – one cow per poor family). He reported that maize bran is the most contaminated ingredients being used to produce feedstuffs (Minagri, 2018).

## Aflatoxin ($M_1$) in Milk

Occurrence of aflatoxin $M_1$ in milk and its products is increasingly reported. In some samples, especially those obtained from Asian countries, $AFM_1$ concentration was higher than the limit of 0.05 µg/l imposed by many countries (Kaleibar and Helan, 2013; Chohan *et al.*, 2016). In an investigation made in India by Rastogi *et al.* (2004), it was found that 87% of liquid milk were found to be contaminated with $AFM_1$ ranging from 28-164 µg/l. Almost 99% of the contaminated samples exceeded the European communities (EC) limit (Rastogis *et al.*, 2004). Henry *et al.* (2004) reported a similar upsurge of contaminated milk with $AFM_1$ in Indonesia, Philippines and Thailand. However, in some European countries, relatively low levels of aflatoxin $M_1$ were determined in mild samples (Trucksers, 2006). Those differences may be related to the stringent regulation of aflatoxin $B_1$ in complementary feedstuffs for dairy cattle in European countries (Kamkar *et al.*, 2011). Several authors have reported that higher concentration of $AFM_1$ in cold seasons as compared to hot seasons (Belandzie *et al.*, 2010). At present many countries have set maximum acceptable levels for $AFM_1$ in milk and dairy products. USFDA has set the aflatoxin $M_1$ permissive level in milk upto 0.5 µg/kg while African, Asian and some European countries have their limit of 0.05µg/kg.

Bakirci *et al.*, 2001 in his work investigated the levels of $AFM_1$ in the dairy products made from contaminated milk (butter, butter milk, cream & skimmed milk). The mean aflatoxin $M_1$ level found in cream samples was 64.4% high compared to bulk-tank milk, whereas, mean $AFM_1$ level of skim milk was 3% higher than those of bulk-tank milk. Direct correlation between $AFB_1$ consumption and $AFM_1$ excretion in milk and urine samples has been observed. Through the breast milk with $AFM_1$ nursing mothers can provide a source of aflatoxin exposure to infant (El-Nezami, 1995). In general, the $AFM_1$ concentration in milk is dependent on following factors.

### Animal Type

Van Egmond (1989) reported that excreted amount of $AFM_1$ in the milk of dairy cow was 1-2% of ingested $AFB_1$. On the other hand, the carry over rates for mares (0.04 - 0.05%), ewes (0.60 to 0.72%) and goats (2.5 to 2.7%) have been reported. For mares producing milk upto 3kg/day, the carry over rate ranged between 0.04- 0.05%, which is more than 10 fold lower when compared to common daily cattle (Battacone *et al.*, 2003).

## Milking Day (Even from One Milking to the Next)

Day after the $AFM_1$ containing ration was fed and milk toxin failed to be detected five days after the feeding program was discontinued. $AFM_1$ can be found in milk within 12 – 24 h after the first ingestion of $AFM_1$ (Battacone *et al.*, 2003) and increased as soon as the first milking after animal ingestion with a pattern of increment up between 7th and 12th days of $AFM_1$ ingestion (Masoero *et al.*, 2007). In a related study, dairy cows in the early lactation stage (2 – 4 weeks) and in late lactation weeks (34 – 36 weeks) were fed with $AFM_1$ contaminated feed. The early lactation phase had $AFM_1$ excretion in milk upto 6.2% while it delivered to 1.8% in the late lactation stages (Veldman *et al.*, 1992).

**Milk Yield:** Masoero has suggested that milk yield is one of the major factors affecting the total excretion of $AFM_1$ (Masoero *et al.*, 2007). Dairy cows with high yielding races have comparatively high (6.2%) carry over rate of $AFM_1$ (Veldman *et al.*, 1992).

**Seasons:** A number of studies have shown that the mean contamination level of $AFM_1$ in autumn and winter (cold season) was significantly higher than those of spring and summer (Rashmi *et al.*, 2009); Tajkarimi *et al.*, 2008; Heinonen *et al.*, 1996; Bakirci, 2001). This might be due to the fact the fully harvested grass, pasture, weed and rough feed were found more commonly in spring and summer than in winter (Galvano *et al.*, 1996; Celi *et al.*, 2005). Takar and Vengust (2008) reported that in winter cows are fed with greater amount of compound feeds, which exceed the allowed $AFB_1$ content.

## Transmission (Carry-over of Aflatoxin)

A number of nutritional and physiological factors such as feeding ration routine, ingestion rate, digestion potential, animals health status, hepatic biotransformation capabilities and lactation efficiency influence the extent of aflatoxin transfer from feed to milk referred as carryover. Carryover rate also varies from one milking to the next milking stages of the cattle. In high-yielding cows, the consumption of significantly higher amounts of concentrated feeds might result in carry-over percentages as high as 6-2% (Veldmal *et al.*, 1992). Statutory limits have been defined for animal feeds (including feeds for dairy cows) in order to avoid transfer of toxins from feed to milk. The legislation set for aflatoxin contamination in cattle feed of lactating animals need to be monitored whether it is sufficient to maintain the threshold level (0.05 µg/kg) of $AFM_1$ in milk.

Aflatoxin $M_1$ is considered to be the major metabolite excreted with milk in dairy cows and other ruminants. In addition, aflatoxin $M_2$ and $M_4$, originating from hepatic - biotransformation reaction of other natural aflatoxins, have been found to be excreted with milk, however, at very low amounts. The hydroxyl derivative of $AFB_1$ – aflatoxicol is also excreted with milk (Carvajal *et al.*, 2003).

## Control of Aflatoxin in Cattle Feed and Milk

The economic consequences of aflatoxins and its potential health problem to human beings have created an urgent need to eliminate or at least control aflatoxin contaminated of food and feed. Several approaches towards the control of aflatoxin contamination have been summarized by different investigators (CAST, 1989; Robens and Richard, 1992; Sinha and Bhatnagar, 1998; Scott, 1998; Choudhary and Kumari, 2010).

Some of the most critical approaches for management of aflatoxins are to avoid or minimize the most susceptible feed raw materials viz. coconut cakes, maize, cotton seed cakes and rice flour etc.). In addition, regular survey, analytical control of feed ingredient, sorting and screening of feed stuffs removal of contaminated feeds etc need to be implemented rigorously. In case, weather conditions are conducive for mould growth and the grains sources exhibiting the chances of contamination of feed stuffs, the $AFM_1$ contamination of milk produce needs to be screened prior being dairy processing as because of the safety point of view. A linear relationship between the amount of $AFM_1$ in milk and $AFB_1$ in feed consumed by the animals has been reported (Bakirci, 2001). Therefore the emphasis has been on reduction or removal of $AFB_1$ from feedstuffs with consequent diminutions of $AFM_1$ from milk.

The most effective way to control $AFM_1$ in liquid milk and dairy products is to prevent the initial contamination of feeds consumed by dairy cattle. For this purpose, specific regulations for feed exist in many countries (FAO, 2003). A code of practice for reducing $AFB_1$ in raw materials has been developed by the cedex committee on food additives and contaminants (Van Ergmond, 1994). Good manufacturing practices (GMP) and good storage practices which reduce $AFB_1$ in feed stuffs through reduction in mould growth are applicable. If such methods fail to reduce $AFB_1$ formation, other chemical, physical or biological methods can be applied. At high-pressure and high-temperature (80°C – 100°C for 20-60 minutes) ammonization (0.5 – 2%) eliminate $AFB_1$ from feed and subsequently, $AFM_1$ in milk. Alkaline heat treatment, or nixtamalization, which is used traditionally in the treatment of maize for the manufacture of tortillas, significantly reduced the concntration of aflatoxins in feed.

Several other methods such as Physical methods (irradiation), extraction by alkaline solvents, absorption by sequestering agents or heat treatments have showed different levels of aflatoxins reduction in feed. Activated carbon and montmorillonite clays effectively bind $AFB_1$ *in vitro* (Galvano *et al.*, 2001; Huwig *et al.*, 2001). Biological methods can also be used to eliminate aflatoxins. Microbial treatment of feedstuffs with *Flavobacterium auranthiacum* has been reported to degrade aflatoxin (JECFA, 2000). Application of non-aflatoxigenic biocompetitive, native *A. flavus* strains to outcompete toxigenic isolates in the fields has been found effective in significantly reducing aflatoxins contamination (Cotty *et al.*, 1994). Filamentous fungus *Trichoderma* sp. has been accepted as the most potential biological control agent for fungal control (Bilgrami and Choudhary 1989; Inglis and Kawchuk, 2002). They reported that two isolates of *Trichiderma harzianum* and two of *T. viride* inhibited the growth of *A. flavus*. *Trichoderma viride* is capable of inhibiting the production of $AFB_1$ (73.5%) and aflatoxin $G_1$ to 100% when it is being co-cultured with *Aspergillus flavus* (Choudhary, 1992).

Activated carbon, sodium bentonite and esterified glucomannan have shown to reduce transfer of $AFM_1$ into milk (31-65%) (Diaz *et al.*, 2003). It was reported that by supplementing sodium bentonite and activated charcoal by 1% for early lactating goats resulted in significant reduction of $AFM_1$ content of milk and the carryover of aflatoxin from feed to milk, however, causing without any change in the composition of milk (Chopra, 2000).

$AFM_1$ elimination from naturally contaminated milk was reported through Potassium sulphate ($K_2SO_3$) and physical adsorption of the toxin using bentonite. The chemical detoxification/ elimination of $AFM_1$ by applying chemicals with 0.05M Potassium sulphide ($K_2SO_3$) at 25°C for 5 hours was upto 46%, however, this was as high as 89% when 0.4gm of Bentonite per 20 ml of new milk treated for 1 hour (at 25°C) (Applebaum and Marth, 1982). Possible mechanism for degradation of $AFM_1$ by $K_2SO_3$ may involve reactions between the toxin and the bisulphate radical ($HSO_3$). Use of hydrogen peroxide has also been examined to inactivate $AFM_1$ in naturally or artificially contaminated milk under different conditions of temperature and time. Treatment of milk with $H_2O_2$ (0.05%) and exposed with UV light resulted in 89.1% decline in $AFM_1$. However, there was only 60.7% reduction in $AFM_1$ in $H_2O_2$ free milk treated with UV-light (Yousef and Marth, 1989). In a related study, the use of $H_2O_2$ plus riboflavin (30 C, 30 min) followed by heating at 630°C for 30 mins resulted in 98% reduction of the $AFM_1$ present in raw milk.

Chapter 3

# Results

## A. Qualitative and Quantitative Estimations of Aflatoxin from Cattle Feed, Milk and Milk Products

### A.1 Aflatoxin in Cattle Feed

Altogether eight fungal genera were detected and isolated from the collected samples. The spectrum of moulds included *Aspergillus, Fusarium, Penicillium, Rhizopus, Alternaria, Curvularia, Cladosporium* and *Mucor* spp. The incidence of moulds were recorded and their diversity were observed varying with the agro-climatic change of different seasons. Maximum incidence (87%) of *A. flavus* was observed in the monsoons followed by summer (76%). Winters, however, showed the least occurrence of *A. flavus* (19%). Moisture contents in the samples during those periods ranged from16 to 46%, which varied considerable with the seasons and also with the nature of samples.

**Table 6:** Season wise survey of fungi associated in cattle feed samples

| Season | Moisture content | Fungi isolated | % of positive incidence |
|---|---|---|---|
| Winter | 24-32% | *Fusarium monoliforme* | 72 |
| | | *Aspergillus flavus* | 19 |
| | | *A. ochraceus* | 17 |
| | | *Rhizopus stolonifer* | 14 |
| | | *A. candidus* | 11 |
| | | *F. oxysporum* | 27 |
| | | *F. equisetti* | 46 |
| | | *Cladosporium herbarum* | 7 |
| | | *Aspergillus flavus* | 76 |
| | | *A. niger* | 21 |
| | | *A. fumigatus* | 4 |

| | | | |
|---|---|---|---|
| Summer | 16-21% | *Fusarium equisetti* | 17 |
| | | *Penicillium citrinum* | 6 |
| | | *P. chrysogenum* | 5 |
| | | *Rhizopus nigricans* | 13 |
| | | *R. stolonifer* | 12 |
| Monsoon | 34-46% | *Aspergillus flavus* | 87 |
| | | *A. niger* | 27 |
| | | *A. candidus* | 3 |
| | | *A. sydowii* | 2 |
| | | *Penicillium islandicum* | 3 |
| | | *Curvularia lunata* | 19 |
| | | *Alternaria tenuis* | 18 |
| | | *Fusarium monoliforme* | 15 |
| | | *F. acuminatum* | 4 |
| | | *Mucor* sp. | 6 |

Out of 1130 cattle feed samples collected, 381 included commercial feeds, 390 fresh feeds and 359 were from household stored feeds. 753 samples (66.6% of the total samples collected) were observed to be contaminated with $AFB_1$. While considering season-wise incidence of contamination, it was observed that 390 cattle feed samples were collected during winters which included 143 from commercial feeds, 117 from fresh feeds and 130 from household stored feeds. During the summers, 383 cattle feed samples were collected which comprised of 132, 136 and 115 from commercial feeds, fresh feed and household stored feeds, respectively. However, during wet seasons 357 cattle feed samples were collected enlisting 106, 137 and 114 as commercial feeds, fresh feeds and household stored feeds. Maximum amount of aflatoxin $B_1$ (5.02 ± 2.46 µg/kg) [Table -7] was observed in cattle feed samples collected from household stored feeds. Amount of toxins was found significantly high ($p<0.05\%$) compared to commercial or fresh feed samples. 33% of household stored feeds contained aflatoxin $B_1$ level higher than the upper limit of European Union (EU). In a combined observation considering different samples and various seasons in concert, the maximum aflatoxin $B_1$ level was observed in household stored cattle feeds during wet seasons with a mean value of 7.79 ± 2.07 µg/kg [Table- 7, Fig -3] which was followed by commercially available feeds (Mean value 5.17 ± 0.75 µg/kg).The mean value of aflatoxin $B_1$was 3.04 ± 0.68µg/kg in fresh cattle feed. During winters, comparatively lower level of aflatoxin $B_1$ (1.1 ± 0.34 µg/kg) was observed in freshly harvested cattle feed. However, during the summer days maximum contamination of aflatoxin was found in commercial feed with a mean value of 4.34 ± 0.37 µg/kg followed by mean value of household stored cattle feeds (4.22 ± 0.6 µg/kg). Compiling the above findings, it was found that the freshly harvested cattle feeds were relatively secured for cattle consumption as 83-95% of the samples were observed containing aflatoxin level below the EU limit (0.05µg/kg).

**Table 7:** Aflatoxin $B_1$ contamination of cattle feeds in different seasons.

| Season | Number of Samples | | % contaminated samples | Range of Aflatoxin B1 | Mean value of Aflatoxin B1 | Above EU limit (%) |
|---|---|---|---|---|---|---|
| | Screened for aflatoxin | Aflatoxin B1 contaminated Samples | | | | |
| Commercial feed | | | | | | |
| Winter | 143 | 86 | 60.14 | 0.85 - 6.1 | 3.08 ± 1.75 | 15 (17.44) |
| Summer | 132 | 91 | 68.94 | 3.4 - 4.6 | 4.34 ± 0.37 | 21 (23.07) |
| Monsoon | 106 | 78 | 73.58 | 3.6 - 7.56 | 5.17 ± 0.75 | 23 (29.5) |
| Total | 381 | 255 | 66.93 | 0.85 - 7.56 | 4.19 ± 1.05 | 59 (23.33) |
| Fresh Feed | | | | | | |
| Winter | 117 | 70 | 59.83 | 1.5 - 2.6 | 1.1 ± 0.34 | 5 (7.14) |
| Summer | 136 | 82 | 60.29 | 2.8 - 3.8 | 2.04 ± 0.73 | 9 (10.97) |
| Monsoon | 137 | 94 | 68.61 | 3.4 - 4.4 | 3.04 ± 0.68 | 17 (18.1) |
| Total | 390 | 246 | 63.08 | 1.5 - 4.4 | 2.06 ± 0.97 | 31 (12.1) |
| Household feed | | | | | | |
| Winter | 130 | 88 | 67.69 | 1.28 - 3.9 | 3.07 ± 0.82 | 18 (20.45) |
| Summer | 115 | 79 | 68.70 | 2.6 - 4.6 | 4.22 ± 0.6 | 26 (32.9) |
| Monsoon | 114 | 85 | 74.56 | 5.4 - 11.2 | 7.79 ± 2.07 | 39 (45.9) |
| Total | 359 | 252 | 70.19 | 1.2 - 11.2 | 5.02 ± 2.46 | 83 (33.08) |

At p value < 0.05, for season, the mean data for incidence of aflatoxin showed significant difference between winters and monsoons for all three localities under observation. For statistical analysis of Season X Feed, CD is 2.08 (at 5%) which clearly showed that during summer and monsoon the mean value of aflatoxin was significantly higher compared to winter. In case of feeds procured from commercial centres and household, showed significantly higher level of aflatoxin $B_1$ compared to fresh feed.

### A.1.1 Aflatoxin $B_1$ in Different Types of Cattle Feeds

The mean value of aflatoxin $B_1$ content in commercial cattle feed samples was 4.19 ± 1.05µg/kg which ranged from 0.85µg/kg to 7.56µg/kg with 23.3% of samples beyond the acceptable limit (0.05µg/kg) of European Union. The mean value of aflatoxin recorded in the household cattle feed was 5.02 ± 2.46µg/kg, ranging from 1.2µg/ kg to 11.2µg/ kg. Comparatively, freshly reaped feeds showed the least amount of aflatoxin content in consideration to the three sources of cattle feeds. The mean value of the aflatoxin $B_1$ content in fresh cattle feed was 2.06 ± 0.97µg/kg where range of aflatoxin $B_1$content was found 1.5 µg/ kg to 4.4 µg/ kg with 12.1 % of feed samples above EU acceptable limit. The records thus obtained showed that the cattle fed with fresh feed bear less chance of poisoning with aflatoxin. It is evident from Fig. 3 that freshly harvested feeds were comparatively safe for the cattle consumption even during monsoon days as 83% of samples were within the EU limit.

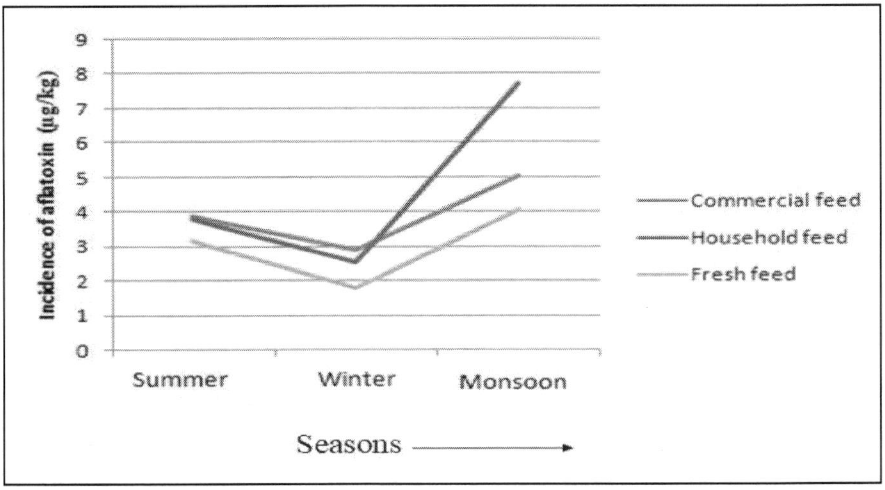


**Fig. 3:** Aflatoxin contamination in various cattle feeds

CD value for types of cattle feeds at 5% = 2.08.

At $p<0.05$, the mean value of $AFB_1$ in household and commercial feed was significantly high compared to fresh feed.

### A.1.2 Aflatoxin $B_1$ in Different Seasons

Considerable impact of seasons was observed on aflatoxin $B_1$ content in various cattle feeds. During monsoons, there was significantly high level of ($p<0.05$) of aflatoxin contamination in different types of feeds of cattle (Fig - 4) obtained from different locations.

The mean level of contamination of aflatoxin during the dry and cold seasons was 3.53µg/kg and 2.55 µg/kg, respectively showing non-significant (Fig - 5) differences between the mean levels of aflatoxins during summers and winters.

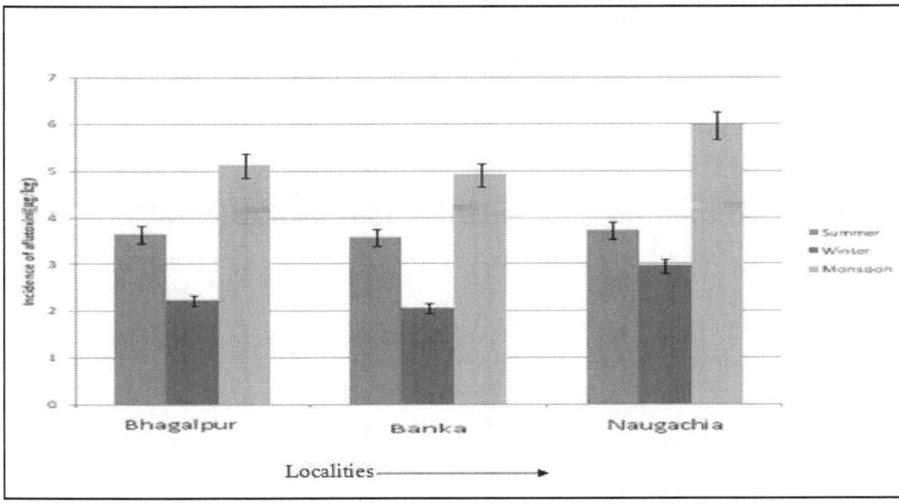


**Fig. 4:** Aflatoxin $B_1$ levels in cattle feed of different seasons.

CD value for season at 5% was 2.08

At $p<0.05$, the mean value of aflatoxin $B_1$ incidence during wet season was significantly higher compared to winter. However, the mean value of $AFB_1$ incidence during summer was at par with the winter.

### A.1.3 Aflatoxin $B_1$ Contamination at Different Districts

Among the localities, the feed samples obtained from Naugachia recorded the maximum mean level of aflatoxin in every season. The mean value of aflatoxin level in cattle feed of Naugachia was 4.2 ± 1.56µg/kg followed by Bhagalpur (3.7 ± 1.45µg/kg) and Banka (3.5 ± 1.43) [Fig -4]. During wet seasons cattle feed of Naugachia contained considerably higher (11.14µg/kg) level of toxin.

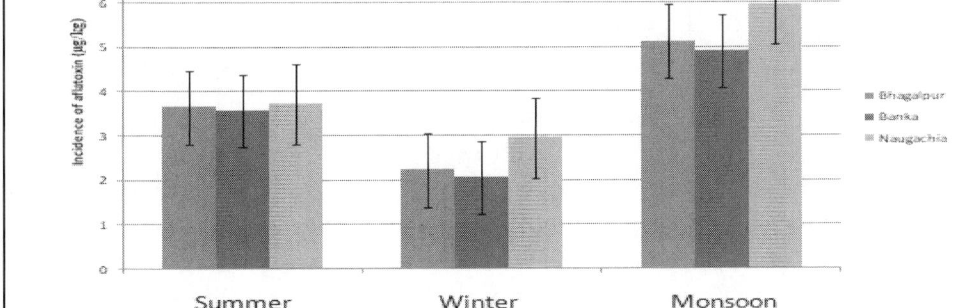


**Fig. 5:** Levels of aflatoxin $B_1$ contamination at different localities

CD value for season at 5% is 2.08

At $p<0.05$, the mean value of aflatoxin $B_1$ incidence during wet season was significantly higher compared to winter. However, the mean value of $AFB_1$ incidence during summer was at par with the winter considering any type of cattle feed.

## A.2 Aflatoxin Contamination in Milk and Milk Products

The results obtained by the qualitative and quantitative analysis of aflatoxin $M_1$ from different milk and milk products are shown in Table - 8. The study revealed that the per cent contamination of aflatoxin $M_1$ depends upon the type of milk and milk products. We examined a total of 182 samples of milk and milk products among which 75 (41.1%) were found contaminated with aflatoxin $M_1$.

**Table 8:** Aflatoxin M1 contamination in different milk samples and milk products

| Different milk and milk product | No. of samples | No. of positive samples | >0.5 µg/kg | >0.05 ug/kg | Range of aflatoxin $M_1$ (µg/kg) | Mean ± SD |
|---|---|---|---|---|---|---|
| Cow milk | 25 | 14(58) | 1 | 9 | 0.011- 0.156 | 0.076 ± 0.046 |
| Buffalo milk | 23 | 12 (52.1) | 0 | 6 | 0.020 - 0.22 | 0.073±0.062 |
| Goat milk | 9 | 3(33.3) | 0 | 2 | 0.023- 0.072 | 0.045±0.025 |
| Sudha dairy milk | 8 | 2 (25) | 0 | 0 | 0.010-0.016 | 0.013±0.004 |
| Milk powder | 8 | 3 (37.5) | 0 | 0 | 0.009 - 0.024 | 0.013±0.012 |
| Curd | 20 | 9 (45) | 0 | 4 | 0.016- 0.102 | 0.046± 0.029 |
| Khoya | 13 | 7 (53.8) | 0 | 4 | 0.025- 0.118 | 0.060± 0.035 |
| Paneer | 23 | 8 (34.7) | 0 | 1 | 0.013- 0.054 | 0.032±0.015 |
| Cheese | 12 | 3 (25) | 0 | 0 | 0.00- 0.022 | 0.013±0.012 |
| Rabri | 24 | 8 (33.3) | 0 | 2 | 0.017- 0.92 | 0.043±0.024 |
| Ice-cream | 10 | 4 (40) | 0 | 0 | 0.007- 0.031 | 0.018±0.010 |
| Milk shake | 7 | 2 (28.5) | 0 | 0 | 0.005- 0.023 | 0.014±0.013 |
| **Total** | **182** | **75 (41.1%)** | **1** | **28** | **0.00 - 0.156** | **0.037 ± 0.023** |

At p value $< 0.05$, for the quantitative incidence of $AFM_1$ in the milk and milk products, the mean data showed significant difference between raw milk of cows, buffaloes and goats to that of Sudha dairy milk, milk powder and milk shake for all three localities under observation. For statistical analysis of one way variance of milk and milk products, CD (at 5%) which clearly showed remarkable difference of $AFM_1$ incidence in raw milk to that of processed milk products.

In case of milk samples, maximum contamination (58%) occurred in cow milk samples followed by buffalo milk (52%) however, minimum contamination (25%)

of aflatoxin $M_1$ was observed in Sudha milk (25%). Among the milk products, maximum (53.8%) contamination was observed in local made product khoya followed by curd (45%). Cheese and milkshakes were less contaminated by aflatoxin $M_1$, 25% and 28.5%, respectively.

The quantitative analysis of aflatoxin $M_1$ revealed that range of aflatoxin was high in buffalo milk (0.020-0.22µg/kg) followed by cow milk samples (0.011-0.156µg/kg). Out of 182 samples tested, 28 samples contained toxin in the range of 0.05µg/kg to 0.5µg/kg. However, one sample (cow milk) was highly contaminated with aflatoxin, the level exceeding 0.5µg/kg. The remaining 46 samples were contaminated by aflatoxin $M_1$ but the quantity was less than 0.05µg/kg. USFDA has set a maximum permissible level for aflatoxin $M_1$ of 0.5µg/Kg (in milk), however, in Europe and in some African and Asian countries, the maximum acceptable level of aflatoxin $M_1$ in milk is 0.05µg/kg. In order to maintain this level, it is desirable that the aflatoxin $B_1$ level in feeds of dairy animals must be limited to keep the levels of $AFM_1$ in milk < 0.05µg/Kg.

Mean concentrations of aflatoxin $M_1$ in different milk and milk products were also determined. In our studies cow (0.076µg/kg) and buffalo milk (0.073µg/kg) samples contained comparatively high $AFM_1$ concentration.

### A.2.1 Regional Variations of Aflatoxin $M_1$ Among Different Milk Samples

Regional variations in aflatoxin $M_1$ contamination of milk of different cattle (cows, buffaloes and goats) were also analysed. Aflatoxin $M_1$ contaminations in milk of different cattle of urban, semi-urban and rural areas were monitored (Table - 9). Considering all types of cattle, maximum contamination (58%) of aflatoxin $M_1$ occurred in milk of urban areas cow milk followed by buffalo (52%) and goat milk (48). In semi-urban areas, the contamination of aflatoxin $M_1$ was comparatively less than urban areas, where 48% of buffalo milk samples, 46% of cow milk samples and 36% of goat milk samples were positive to aflatoxin contamination. However, in the milk samples of rural areas per cent contamination was comparatively less than semi urban and urban area where 36% samples in milk from buffaloes were positive to aflatoxin $AFM_1$ followed by 32% from cow and goat. However, maximum concentration of aflatoxin $M_1$ was obtained in buffalo milk of urban areas (mean = 0.126µg/kg) followed by cow milk of urban areas (0.105µg/kg).

**Table 9:** Regional variations of aflatoxin $M_1$ in milk samples of different cattle

| Species | Region | Positive sample (%) | Mean ± SD |
|---|---|---|---|
| Cow | Urban | 58 | 0.105 ± 0.192 |
| | Semi-urban | 46 | 0.074 ± 0.112 |
| | Rural | 32 | 0.038 ± 0.036 |
| Buffalo | Urban | 52 | 0.126 ± 0.261 |
| | Semi-urban | 48 | 0.102 ± 0.222 |
| | Rural | 36 | 0.031 ± 0.028 |

| Goat | Urban | 48 | 0.033 ± 0.021 |
|---|---|---|---|
| | Semi-urban | 36 | 0.035 ± 0.022 |
| | Rural | 32 | 0.032 ± 0.017 |

### A.2.2 Seasonal Variations in Aflatoxin $M_1$

Table - 10 shows the seasonal variation of aflatoxin contamination in milk of different cattle (cow, buffalo and goat). The observation revealed that the aflatoxin $M_1$ contamination was significantly high in monsoons and spring seasons compared to winter season. In wet seasons, out of 70 samples of cow milk 32 (45.7%) were contaminated with aflatoxin $M_1$ followed by 28 (42.4%) of buffalo milk samples, however, in goat milk the per cent of contamination (35.2%) was less than cow and buffalo. In spring, out of 65 samples of cow milk, 22 samples (33.8%) contained aflatoxin $M_1$ which, however, was higher than buffalo milk in which out of 54 samples, 17 (31.4%) contained aflatoxin $M_1$.

Among different seasons, winter milk samples of different cattle milk showed less contamination than spring, summer and monsoons. During those seasons, cow milk contamination rate was higher than buffalo and goat milk. 21.4% and 25% of buffalo milk were contaminated in winter and summer, respectively. Per cent of aflatoxin positive samples was significantly low in goat milk than cow and buffalo milk.

**Table 10:** Seasonal variations of aflatoxin $M_1$ in milk samples of different seasons

| Season | Species | Total no. of sample | Positive sample (%) | Range of aflatoxin $M_1$ | | | Mean |
|---|---|---|---|---|---|---|---|
| | | | | 0.5 µg/kg | 0.05 to 0.5µg/kg | □0.05 µg/kg | |
| Spring | Cow | 65 | 22 (33.8) | 2 | 7 | 13 | 0.137±0 .193 |
| | Buffalo | 54 | 17 (31.4) | 3 | 8 | 6 | 0.177± 0.227 |
| | Goat | 29 | 6 (20.6) | 0 | 2 | 4 | 0.038± 0.027 |
| Summer | Cow | 104 | 32 (30.7) | 3 | 12 | 17 | 0.128±0.175 |
| | Buffalo | 96 | 24 (25) | 2 | 13 | 9 | 0.099±0.146 |
| | Goat | 40 | 7 (17.5) | 0 | 2 | 5 | 0.036± 0.027 |
| Monsoon | Cow | 70 | 32 (45.7) | 4 | 18 | 10 | 0.143± 0.217 |
| | Buffalo | 66 | 28 (42.4) | 2 | 9 | 17 | 0.100±0.198 |
| | Goat | 17 | 6 (35.2) | 0 | 1 | 5 | 0.041±0.020 |
| Winter | Cow | 92 | 25 (27.1) | 0 | 6 | 19 | 0.034± 0.021 |
| | Buffalo | 84 | 18 (21.4) | 0 | 7 | 11 | 0.039± 0.025 |
| | Goat | 41 | 15 (26.5) | 0 | 0 | 15 | 0.015± 0.012 |

At p value < 0.05, for the quantitative incidence of $AFM_1$ in the milk of cattle, the mean data showed significant difference between raw milk obtained during winter season to any other seasons (summer, spring, monsoons). For statistical analysis of Season X milk, CD was 0.0343 (at 5%) which clearly showed that milk obtained during spring, summer and monsoons, the mean value of aflatoxin was significantly higher compared to winter.

Table - 10 also evidenced the variation in the level of aflatoxin concentration in milk of different cattle (cow, buffalo and goat). It was observed that the concentration of aflatoxin $M_1$ was high during the spring season (fig- 6, 7). In this season mean value of $M_1$ concentration was maximum in buffalo (0.177µg/kg) followed by cow milk samples (0.137µg/kg), however, the mean value was the lowest in goat milk samples (0.038µg/kg). In this season two cow milk samples (out of 22 samples) were grouped in the category in which the concentration exceeded 0.5µg/kg, however, 7 samples came under the range between the 0.5µg/kg to 0.05µg/kg and rest 13 samples concentration was less than 0.05µg/kg. In case of buffalo milk, out of 17 samples, concentration of aflatoxin $M_1$ in 3 samples were more than 0.5µg/kg, 8 in the range of 0.5µg/kg to 0.05µg/kg, 6 samples contained concentration less than 0.05µg/kg. However, out of 6 positive samples of goat, 2 in between the range of 0.5µg/kg to 0.05µg/kg and in 4 samples aflatoxin $M_1$ contamination was less than 0.05µg/kg.

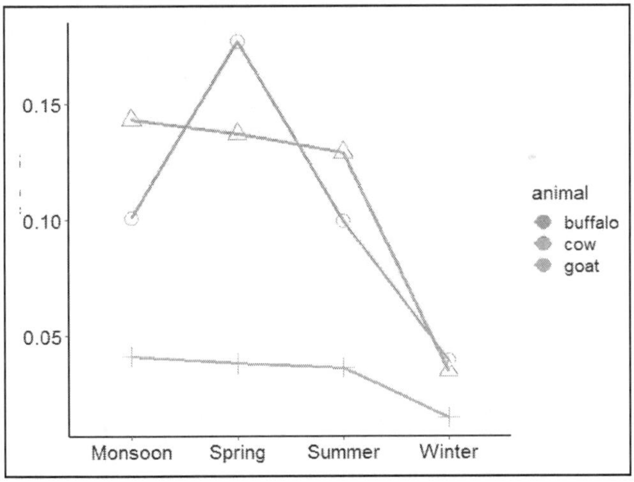


**Fig. 6:** Mean aflatoxin $M_1$ contamination among milk samples of different cattle and seasons

At p<0.05, the mean value of $AFM_1$ in milk obtained from three cattles generated a CD value of 0.0524. The critical difference clearly showed that the mean value $AFM_1$ incidence in milk obtained from cows and buffaloes were highly significant compared to goat milk.

In the summer, mean value of $M_1$ concentration was maximum in cow milk (0.128µg/kg) which was more than buffalo milk samples (0.099µg/kg), however, the mean value was low in goat milk samples (0.036µg/kg). Out of 32 cow milk samples of this season, 3 samples contained the level exceeding 0.5µg/kg, however 12 samples had fallen in the range between 0.5µg/kg to 0.05µg/kg and rest 17 samples had less than 0.05µg/kg of aflatoxin $M_1$. In case of buffalo milk, out of 24 positive samples, concentration of 2 samples were more than 0.5µg/kg, 13 in between the range of 0.5µg/kg to 0.05µg/kg and 9 samples had the amount less than 0.05µg/kg. However, out of 7 positive samples of goat milk, 2 were in the range of 0.5µg/kg to 0.05µg/kg and 5 samples concentration of aflatoxin $M_1$ less than 0.05µg/kg.

In the monsoon, mean value of $M_1$ concentration was maximum in cow milk (0.143µg/kg) which was followed by buffalo milk samples (0.100µg/kg) and the mean value was minimum in goat milk samples (0.041µg/kg). In this season 4 cow milk samples (out of 32 positive samples) were grouped in the category of exceeding the regulation limit of 0.5µg/kg, however 18 samples were in the range of 0.5µg/kg to 0.05µg/kg and rest in 10 samples the amount of toxin was less than 0.05µg/kg. In case of buffalo milk, out of 28 positive samples, 2 contained more than 0.5µg/kg, 9 had fallen in the range of 0.5µg/kg to 0.05µg/kg, in 17 samples contamination level was less than 0.05µg/kg. However, out of the 6 positive samples of goat, only one sample could fall in the range of 0.5µg/kg to 0.05µg/kg and in 5 samples concentration of aflatoxin $M_1$ was less than 0.05µg/kg.

In winter, the concentration of aflatoxin $M_1$ was the lowest than other seasons. In this season mean value of $M_1$ concentration was maximum in buffalo milk (0.039µg/kg) where, it was more than cow milk samples (0.034µg/kg) and mean value was minimum in goat milk samples (0.015µg/kg). In this season six cow milk samples (out of 25 positive samples) were grouped in the category in which concentration was in between the 0.5µg/kg to 0.05µg/kg and rest in 19 samples, the concentration was less than 0.05µg/kg. In case of buffalo milk, out of 18 positive samples, 11 was in the range of 0.5µg/kg to 0.05µg/kg, in 7 samples concentration was less than 0.05µg/kg. However, out of 15 positive samples of goat milk, concentrations of aflatoxin $M_1$ of all samples were less than 0.05µg/kg.

The mean value of aflatoxin $M_1$ was found maximum in spring which was highly significant as compared to winter but was at par with summer and monsoon (Fig - 6). However, during the spring, summer and monsoon there were non-significant differences with respect to the levels of aflatoxin $M_1$. Mean value of aflatoxin $M_1$ in winter season was 0.030µg/ kg which was significantly different from other three seasons (spring, summer and monsoon). Minimum value of aflatoxin $M_1$ was found in goat milk which was however, significantly low as compared to cow and buffalo. Maximum level of milk toxin was found in cow which, however, was at par with buffalo milk samples.

The analysis of variance with respect to aflatoxin $M_1$ content in milk in different cattles for different seasons differed significantly. F-value for season was found 4.702 whose probability value was 0.001. This reflected the facts that the levels of aflatoxin $M_1$ contamination of different cattle milk (cow, buffalo, goat) was influenced with the seasons. Mean value of aflatoxin $M_1$ level in cow and buffalo were at par which, however, was significantly high from goat milk (Fig- 7).

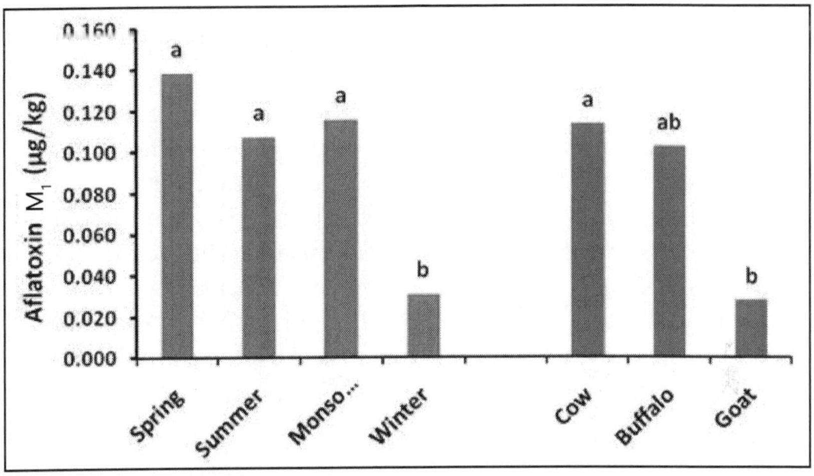


**Fig. 7:** Variations of aflatoxin $M_1$ contamination in the milk of different cattle (cow, buffalo, goat) in different seasons.

At $p<0.05$, the one way analysis of variance of $AFM_1$ incidence in season had a CD value of 0.0343 and that of $AFM_1$ in milk had 0.0524. The CD value among seasons statistically supported the data obtained where the $AFM_1$ incidence in spring, summer and monsoon were highly significant compared to that of winter. The CD value among the cattle further supported the data obtained where the mean value of $AFM_1$ incidence in cows and buffaloes were highly significant compared to that of goat milk.

## B. Carry-over of Aflatoxin $B_1$ from Cow Feed to Milk (as Aflatoxin $M_1$)

The ability of cattle to transform aflatoxin $B_1$ of feed to aflatoxin $M_1$ in the milk has previously been studied by some researchers (Veldman *et al.*, 1992; Masoero *et al.*, 2007; Britzi *et al.*, 2013; Nile *et al.*, 2015). They observed that the carry over rate in the cows (milked twice daily) was 1-2% of aflatoxin $B_1$ in low yielding cows (<20 kg milk yield/ day) and upto 6% in high yielding cows. In previous investigations at abroad it was observed that the carry over rate was directly correlated to the days in lactation and milk yield (Veldman, 1992; Diaz *et al.*, 2004; Masoero *et al.*, 2007). Carry over rate is supposed to be influenced by several other factors viz. species differences, general health of the animal, hepatic biotransformation capacity, alveolar cell permeability, however, those observations need to be substantiated with experimental evidences.

The present study was carried out to determine the carry over rate of aflatoxin $M_1$ in milk of cows of Bhagalpur district in order to determine the acceptable aflatoxin $B_1$ intake in feed. Table - 11 shows the summarized data of twelve cows in early lactation stage and the carry over rate of aflatoxin $M_1$. Early lactating cows were selected which were of the duration of 2-4 weeks (after calving) and same cows while in late lactating period i.e (34 to 36 weeks of lactation) were employed for further experiments (Table - 12). The total mean daily intake of aflatoxin $B_1$ was 42.7 ± 3.6µg. The milk yields of each cow were recorded daily, with the mean of 20.1 ± 1.06kg/day and 11.6 ± 1.39 kg/day for early lactation and late lactation cows, respectively. Aflatoxin $M_1$ excretion during early lactation periods were 2.2µg/day, ranging from 1.7µg/day to 2.6µg/day. The average carry over rate was 0.052% (ranging from 0.038 ± 0.007 to 0.061± 0.011). Remarkable differences were found in the carry over rate of aflatoxin between early lactation to that of late lactation period of milking. While comparing two different lactating periods, the difference of carryover rate was found in a factor of 3.2. Variations among $AFM_1$ excretion were observed among the cows of same stage, however, consuming approximately similar concentrations of $AFB_1$. C1, C2.....C12 indicate the cow numbered for experimental purposes.

**Table 11:** Intake of aflatoxin and its excretion in milk of individual cow during early lactation (two to four weeks after calving).

| Lactation period | Cows | $AFB_1$ intake (µg/ day) (Mean) | Milk yield (kg/ day) (Mean) | $AFM_1$ concentration in milk (µg/kg) (Mean) | $AFM_1$ excretion in milk (µg/day) (Mean) | Carry-over rate (%) |
|---|---|---|---|---|---|---|
| Early lactation (2 - 4 weeks after calving) | C1 | 46.8 ± 0.76 | 19.7 ± 1.44 | 0.07 ± 0.02 | 2.5 ± 0.66 | 0.053 ± 0.009 |
| | C2 | 48.9 ± 1.02 | 19.3 ± 1.36 | 0.05 ± 0.01 | 2.2 ± 0.57 | 0.045 ± 0.008 |
| | C3 | 37.8 ± 1.03 | 21.4 ± 0.82 | 0.06 ± 0.01 | 2.3 ± 0.52 | 0.061 ± 0.011 |
| | C4 | 44.8 ± 1.43 | 19.6 ± 1.41 | 0.04 ± 0.01 | 1.7 ± 0.41 | 0.038 ± 0.007 |
| | C5 | 43.7 ± 0.93 | 20.3 ± 1.2 | 0.06 ± 0.02 | 2.2 ± 0.54 | 0.050 ± 0.009 |
| | C6 | 36.6 ± 1.41 | 18.8 ± 1.11 | 0.05 ± 0.01 | 2.2 ± 0.49 | 0.060 ± 0.011 |
| | C7 | 42.5 ± 0.86 | 19.4 ± 1.37 | 0.05 ± 0.01 | 2.3 ± 0.61 | 0.054 ± 0.009 |
| | C8 | 41.7 ± 1.74 | 21.7 ± 0.95 | 0.04 ± 0.01 | 1.8 ± 0.45 | 0.043 ± 0.008 |
| | C9 | 42.5 ± 0.94 | 18.6 ± 1.09 | 0.06 ± 0.01 | 2.4 ± 0.63 | 0.056 ± 0.010 |
| | C10 | 44.3 ± 1.01 | 20.6 ± 1.27 | 0.07 ± 0.02 | 2.6 ± 0.71 | 0.059 ± 0.011 |
| | C11 | 44.2 ± 0.88 | 19.7 ± 1.36 | 0.05 ± 0.11 | 2.2 ± 0.88 | 0.050 ± 0.009 |
| | C12 | 38.8 ± 1.63 | 21.6 ± 0.91 | 0.04 ± 0.01 | 1.9 ± 0..46 | 0.049 ± 0.009 |
| **Mean** | | **42.7 ± 3.6** | **20.1 ± 1.06** | **0.05 ± 0.01** | **2.2 ± 0.27** | **0.052 ± 0.007** |

**Table 12:** Intake of aflatoxin and its excretion in milk of individual cow during late lactating period (34 to 36 weeks after calving).

| Lactation period | Cows | $AFB_1$ intake (µg/ day) (Mean) | Milk yield (kg/ day) (Mean) | $AFM_1$ concentration in milk (µg/kg) (Mean) | $AFM_1$ excretion in milk (µg/kg) (Mean) | Carry-over rate (%) |
|---|---|---|---|---|---|---|
| Late lactation (34 - 36 weeks after calving) | C1 | 38.7 ± 1.59 | 13.4 ± 0.67 | 0.03 ± 0.02 | 0.9 ± 0.72 | 0.023 ± 0.009 |
| | C2 | 36.9 ± 1.01 | 14.6 ± 1.14 | 0.04 ± 0.02 | 0.7 ± 0.34 | 0.019 ± 0.010 |
| | C3 | 36.4 ± 1.24 | 12.1 ± 0.86 | 0.04 ± 0.01 | 0.7 ± 0.89 | 0.019 ± 0.006 |
| | C4 | 35.8 ± 0.97 | 10.2 ± 1.34 | 0.03 ± 0.01 | 0.6 ± 0.17 | 0.017 ± 0.008 |
| | C5 | 34.9 ± 1.41 | 11.8 ± 1.41 | 0.03 ± 0.02 | 0.4 ± 0.66 | 0.011 ± 0.006 |
| | C6 | 37.2 ± 1.51 | 11.2 ± 1.23 | 0.05 ± 0.03 | 1.0 ± 0.53 | 0.027 ± 0.010 |
| | C7 | 34.6 ± 1.34 | 10.9 ± 0.94 | 0.05 ± 0.02 | 0.5 ± 0.81 | 0.014 ± 0.013 |
| | C8 | 36.8 ± 0.84 | 9.6 ± 1.21 | 0.03 ± 0.02 | 0.3 ± 0.59 | 0.008 ± 0.009 |
| | C9 | 36.4 ± 1.17 | 11.4 ± 1.34 | 0.04 ± 0.01 | 0.4 ± 0.61 | 0.011 ± 0.010 |
| | C10 | 36.9 ± 1.45 | 12.3 ± 1.53 | 0.05 ± 0.01 | 0.7 ± 0.29 | 0.019 ± 0.007 |
| | C11 | 35.7 ± 0.77 | 10.6 ± 1.19 | 0.04 ± 0.03 | 0.5 ± 0.92 | 0.014 ± 0.008 |
| | C12 | 36.2 ± 1.29 | 10.7 ± 0.81 | 0.03 ± 0.01 | 0.4 ± 0.73 | 0.011 ± 0.012 |
| **Mean** | | **36.4 ± 1.08** | **11.6 ± 1.39** | **0.04 ± 0.02** | **0.6 ± 0.21** | **0.016 ± 0.005** |

An average the daily intake of $AFB_1$ during late lactating period was 36.4 ± 1.08µg/day. During late lactation period the yield of milk from same cow decreased (mean 11.6 ± 1.39kg/day) and which eventually resulted into low carry-over of aflatoxin in milk. The mean excretion of $AFM_1$ during late lactation period was 0.6 ± 0.21µg/day (ranging from 0.3 to 1µg/day) with a carry-over rate of 0.016 ± 0.005% (ranging from 0.008 to 0.027). Maximum carry-over rate of 0.061 was found with the intake of 37.8µg/day of $AFB_1$ contaminated feed during early lactating period. However, during late lactating period, maximum carry-over of 0.027 per cent was observed with the ingestion of 37.2µg/day of $AFB_1$ contaminated feed. Aflatoxin $M_1$ carry over within the cattle body has been reported to be influenced by the factors like the amount of aflatoxin $B_1$ absorption from intestinal tract, $AFB_1$ conversion to $AFM_1$ in liver cell, its excretion in urine, bile and milk (Veldman *et al.*, 1992).

Table - 13 and 14 show the data for $AFM_1$ excretion in high and low milk yielding cows of same lactating stage. It was observed that high milk yielding cows showed comparatively higher rate of carry over.

**Table 13:** Intake of aflatoxin and its excretion in the milk of high milk yielding cows.

| | Low intake of $AFB_1$ | | | | | High intake of $AFB_1$ | | | | |
|---|---|---|---|---|---|---|---|---|---|---|
| High milk yielding cows | $AFB_1$ intake (Mean) | Milk yield (kg/day) (Mean) | $AFM_1$ concentration in milk (µg/kg) (Mean) | $AFM_1$ excretion (µg/day) (Mean) | Carry-over rate (%) | $AFB_1$ intake (Mean) | Milk yield (kg/day) (Mean) | $AFM_1$ concentration in milk (µg/kg) (Mean) | $AFM_1$ excretion (µg/day) (Mean) | Carry-over rate (%) |
| Ca | 33 ± 1.24 | 35.5 ± 1.46 | 0.04 ± 0.02 | 1.5 ± 0.56 | 0.045 ± 0.007 | 56 ± 1.37 | 34.2 ± 1.32 | 0.07 ± 0.05 | 2.6 ± 0.64 | 0.046 ± 0.006 |
| Cb | 34 ± 1.52 | 36.2 ± 1.37 | 0.03 ± 0.01 | 1.4 ± 0.49 | 0.041 ± 0.009 | 54 ± 1.56 | 35.4 ± 1.47 | 0.06 ± 0.01 | 2.4 ± 0.49 | 0.044 ± 0.008 |
| Cc | 32 ± 1.67 | 34.6 ± 0.84 | 0.04 ± 0.01 | 1.1 ± 0.89 | 0.034 ± 0.011 | 56 ± 1.74 | 33.6 ± 1.68 | 0.04 ± 0.02 | 1.9 ± 0.81 | 0.034 ± 0.002 |
| Cd | 31 ± 1.23 | 35.8 ± 1.58 | 0.05 ± 0.02 | 1.8 ± 0.46 | 0.058 ± 0.010 | 51 ± 1.67 | 32.5 ± 1.71 | 0.04 ± 0.02 | 2.1 ± 0.56 | 0.041 ± 0.007 |
| Ce | 33 ± 1.81 | 31.9 ± 1.87 | 0.03 ± 0.02 | 1.3 ± 0.67 | 0.039 ± 0.008 | 50 ± 1.81 | 31.1 ± 1.87 | 0.05 ± 0.03 | 1.8 ± 0.79 | 0.036 ± 0.006 |
| Cf | 32 ± 0.94 | 42.6 ± 1.28 | 0.03 ± 0.01 | 0.9 ± 0.75 | 0.028 ± 0.009 | 53 ± 1.79 | 41.7 ± 1.55 | 0.03 ± 0.04 | 1.5 ± 0.82 | 0.028 ± 0.010 |
| Cg | 33 ± 1.37 | 41.8 ± 0.68 | 0.02 ± 0.03 | 1.1 ± 0.88 | 0.033 ± 0.007 | 53 ± 1.25 | 40.9 ± 0.88 | 0.04 ± 0.01 | 2.6 ± 0.61 | 0.049 ± 0.008 |
| Ch | 32 ± 1.84 | 39.4 ± 1.21 | 0.03 ± 0.01 | 1.4 ± 0.51 | 0.044 ± 0.010 | 55 ± 1.39 | 38.8 ± 1.69 | 0.04 ± 0.02 | 2.8 ± 0.57 | 0.051 ± 0.011 |
| Ci | 31 ± 1.44 | 43.7 ± 1.42 | 0.04 ± 0.01 | 1.9 ± 0.64 | 0.061 ± 0.008 | 56 ± 0.89 | 41.8 ± 1.73 | 0.03 ± 0.03 | 3.5 ± 0.87 | 0.063 ± 0.006 |
| Cj | 30 ± 1.31 | 42.6 ± 1.71 | 0.04 ± 0.02 | 1.3 ± 0.79 | 0.043 ± 0.010 | 55 ± 1.41 | 42.1 ± 1.87 | 0.04 ± 0.01 | 2.4 ± 0.71 | 0.044 ± 0.008 |
| Mean Value | 32 ± 1.49 | 38.4 ± 1.44 | 0.04 ± 0.02 | 1.4 ± 0.66 | 0.043 ± 0.009 | 54 ± 1.68 | 37.2 ± 1.61 | 0.04 ± 0.03 | 2.4 ± 0.82 | 0.044 ± 0.009 |

**Table 14:** Intake of aflatoxin and its excretion in the milk of low milk yielding cows.

| | Low intake of $AFB_1$ | | | | | High intake of $AFB_1$ | | | | |
|---|---|---|---|---|---|---|---|---|---|---|
| Low milk yielding cows | $AFB_1$ intake (Mean) | Milk yield (kg/day) (Mean) | $AFM_1$ concentration in milk (µg/kg) (Mean) | $AFM_1$ excretion (µg/day) (Mean) | Carry-over rate (%) | $AFB_1$ intake (Mean) | Milk yield (kg/day) (Mean) | $AFM_1$ concentration in milk (µg/kg) (Mean) | $AFM_1$ excretion (µg/day) (Mean) | Carry-over rate (%) |
| Ck | 32 ± 1.37 | 16.4 ± 1.28 | 0.06 ± 0.06 | 0.9 ± 0.12 | 0.028 ± 0.007 | 54 ± 1.42 | 17.1 ± 1.27 | 0.06 ± 0.02 | 1.6 ± 0.74 | 0.030 ± 0.005 |
| Cl | 32 ± 1.49 | 18.2 ± 1.67 | 0.05 ± 0.04 | 0.8 ± 0.34 | 0.025 ± 0.006 | 53 ± 1.71 | 15.2 ± 1.45 | 0.05 ± 0.02 | 1.5 ± 0.67 | 0.028 ± 0.008 |
| Cm | 33 ± 1.74 | 17.3 ± 1.78 | 0.05 ± 0.07 | 0.7 ± 0.41 | 0.021 ± 0.010 | 54 ± 1.64 | 15.1 ± 1.67 | 0.04 ± 0.03 | 1.3 ± 0.81 | 0.024 ± 0.007 |
| Cn | 32 ± 1.85 | 15.3 ± 1.37 | 0.04 ± 0.05 | 0.8 ± 0.37 | 0.025 ± 0.008 | 54 ± 1.68 | 14.6 ± 0.59 | 0.06 ± 0.01 | 1.1 ± 0.59 | 0.020 ± 0.009 |
| Co | 31 ± 1.67 | 16.1 ± 1.49 | 0.06 ± 0.05 | 0.9 ± 0.28 | 0.029 ± 0.008 | 52 ± 1.49 | 15.3 ± 1.32 | 0.05 ± 0.01 | 1.2 ± 0.28 | 0.023 ± 0.006 |
| Cp | 31 ± 1.49 | 19.4 ± 1.88 | 0.06 ± 0.07 | 1.1 ± 0.51 | 0.035 ± 0.011 | 55 ± 1.81 | 17.8 ± 1.49 | 0.04 ± 0.03 | 1.9 ± 0.37 | 0.035 ± 0.010 |
| Cq | 33 ± 0.87 | 13.5 ± 0.83 | 0.05 ± 0.01 | 0.7 ± 0.48 | 0.021 ± 0.009 | 54 ± 0.88 | 16.2 ± 1.78 | 0.06 ± 0.01 | 1.8 ± 0.71 | 0.033 ± 0.007 |
| Cr | 31 ± 1.78 | 14.9 ± 1.58 | 0.04 ± 0.08 | 0.9 ± 0.34 | 0.029 ± 0.007 | 54 ± 1.38 | 17.1 ± 0.87 | 0.05 ± 0.02 | 2.4 ± 0.88 | 0.044 ± 0.009 |
| Cs | 32 ± 1.51 | 17.1 ± 1.63 | 0.05 ± 0.08 | 1.2 ± 0.29 | 0.038 ± 0.006 | 55 ± 1.65 | 14.2 ± 1.44 | 0.04 ± 0.01 | 2.2 ± 0.73 | 0.040 ± 0.008 |
| Ct | 32 ± 1.87 | 15.4 ± 1.91 | 0.06 ± 0.07 | 1.1 ± 0.39 | 0.034 ± 0.008 | 56 ± 0.79 | 15.6 ± 1.77 | 0.04 ± 0.01 | 1.9 ± 0.67 | 0.034 ± 0.007 |
| Mean value | 31.9 ± 1.66 | 16.4 ± 1.68 | 0.05 ± 0.08 | 0.9 ± 0.38 | 0.029 ± 0.008 | 54 ± 1.68 | 15.8 ± 1.69 | 0.05 ± 0.02 | 1.7 ± 0.77 | 0.031 ± 0.008 |

Maximum carry over rate was 0.063µg/ day, when high milk yielding cows consumed 56µg/day of $AFB_1$ contaminated feed. Rate of carry-over of $AFM_1$, however, varied among high yielding and low yielding cows. The carry-over rate varied by the factor of 1.02 among the high milk yielding cows. In case of low milk yielding cows, the carry-over rate varied by the factor of 1.04. Since the carry over factors were nearly similar and thereby, they supported a linear correlation between the carry-over rate of aflatoxin with milk yield in the same cow (Fig - 8).

The linear correlation has been expressed with the equation: carry-over rate = amount of milk yield per cow per day + 0.013 (r = 0.80). The Figure - 8 clearly shows that at the milk yield of 18.2 kg/day, the carry-over rate was approximately 0.025 which was low than the permissible limit of EU. However, at milk yield of 35.8 and 43.5 kg/day, the carry-over rate was 0.058 and 0.061, respectively which exceeded the regulation limit of EU. EU regulation is based on ALARA (as low as reasonably acceptable level) principle. However, at level 10 times higher than this level (EU limit) is not considered to be harmful for human health (WHO, 2002).

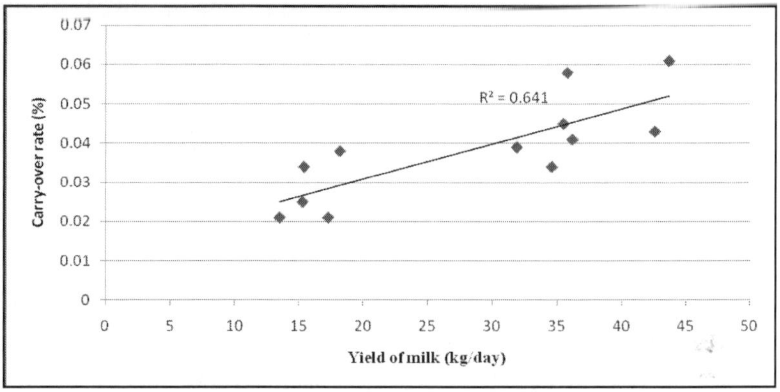


**Fig. 8:** Relationship between milk yield and carry-over rate of aflatoxin

Figure - 9 shows a linear relation between the $AFM_1$ contaminated milk corresponding to the ingestion of $AFB_1$. As evident from the graph that with the evaluation of the amount of $AFB_1$ ingested by the cow, an approximate quantity of the $AFM_1$ content in milk can be predicted, (if other factors such as lactation period, age of the cows etc. remain same). The linear correlation has been expressed with the equation: $AFM_1$ (µg/kg) in milk = amount of $AFB_1$ fed (in µg) per cow per day + 0.001 (r = 0.87).

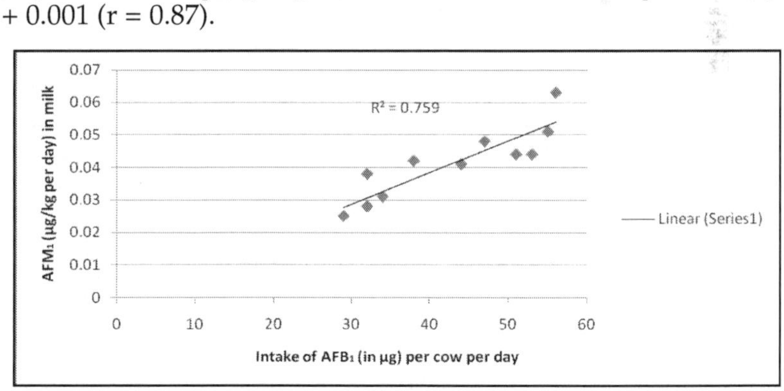


**Fig. 9:** Intake of aflatoxin $B_1$ and secretion of aflatoxin $M_1$ in milk

As evident upto the intake of 47µg/day of aflatoxin $B_1$ in cow feed (TMR = Total Mixed Ration), the aflatoxin $M_1$ excretion remained 0.48 µg/ kg, which was within the EU limit. However, the $AFM_1$ content in milk was found 0.051µg/kg (exceeding EU limit) when the $AFB_1$ intake was 55µg/day. From the equation it can be concluded that average intake of $AFB_1$ for each cow should be less than

55µg per day for the cows of this locality. Maintaining this limit of aflatoxin $B_1$ in feed, the milk safety for human consumption can be maintained.

## C. Influence of Different Variables in the Carryover Rate of Aflatoxin

### C.1 Influence of Localities (Regions) on Carry Over Rate of Aflatoxin

Difference in the carry-over rate was also recorded on the basis of localities such as urban, semi-urban and rural areas of the district. The type and quality of feed given to cows in those areas varied to a large extent. In urban areas, mainly concentrated/ dried feed as wheat straw, paddy straw, wheat bran were provided to the cows. The breeders stacked those dried feeds for months in their store houses. At certain places, household wastes were also found as part of cow feed in urban and semi-urban areas. In semi-urban areas, cows were provided with concentrated/ dried feeds to an extent and also depended upon the reaped grasses of farmlands. However, in rural areas, comparatively higher amounts of fresh green grasses and farmland produce were used. The cattle dwellers in those areas were economically poorer and hence, they were mostly unable to afford commercial cattle feeds. This rendered them to depend upon fresh grasses and farmland wastes which were easily available in villages. Cows were in day time left in grasslands for grazing and they were primarily fed on fresh pastures. Selected cows for this investigation were of first and third lactation (calving cycle) stages of those localities. This was followed in order to maintain the physiological similarity among the test cows.

**Table 15:** Carry-over rate of $AFM_1$ based on the regions (rural, semi-urban and urban) and lactation stages/ calving cycles (first and third lactation).

| Regions | Lactation cycle/ no.of calving of cows | $AFB_1$ intake (µg/day) | Samples tested | Mean milk yield/ day (kg/day) | Mean $AFM_1$ concentration in milk (µg/kg) | Mean $AFM_1$ excretion in milk (µg/day) | Carry-over rate (%) |
|---|---|---|---|---|---|---|---|
| Rural | First | 38.8 ± 1.62 | 20 | 9.8 ± 1.72 | 0.037 ± 0.01 | 1.6 ± 0.52 | 0.039 ± 0.006 |
| Semi Urban | First | 37.4 ± 1.71 | 20 | 10.1 ± 1.81 | 0.041 ± 0.03 | 1.7 ± 0.63 | 0.042 ± 0.007 |
| Urban | First | 42.7 ± 1.43 | 20 | 10.4 ± 1.53 | 0.046 ± 0.04 | 1.9 ± 0.34 | 0.043 ± 0.008 |
| Rural | Third | 41.2 ± 1.49 | 20 | 14.1 ± 1.57 | 0.049 ± 0.02 | 2.4 ± 0.48 | 0.049 ± 0.007 |
| Semi Urban | Third | 42.0 ± 0.91 | 20 | 13.8 ± 1.61 | 0.046 ± 0.03 | 2.1 ± 0.71 | 0.047 ± 0.010 |
| Urban | Third | 40.1 ± 1.84 | 20 | 14.3 ± 1.41 | 0.051 ± 0.02 | 2.3 ± 0.58 | 0.052 ± 0.009 |

Table - 15 revealed the carry-over rate of $AFM_1$ observed in three localities (rural, semi-urban and urban), considering the number of calving/ lactation cycles ($1^{st}$ and $3^{rd}$). In first lactation cycle, the mean average excretion of $AFM_1$ in the milk of rural areas was 0.037 ± 0.01µg/kg (1.6 ± 0.52µg/day). Whereas, for the cows of same lactation period of semi-urban areas, $AFM_1$ excretion was recorded 0.041 ± 0.03µg/kg (1.7 ± 0.63µg/day). However, in the milk of urban cows $AFM_1$ concentration was maximum (0.046 ± 0.04µg/kg; 1.9 ± 0.34µg/day). The carry-over rate of aflatoxin contamination from $AFB_1$ to $AFM_1$ was found slightly higher (0.049 ± 0.008) in urban areas which was followed by semi-urban (0.043 ± 0.007) and rural areas (0.039 ± 0.006).

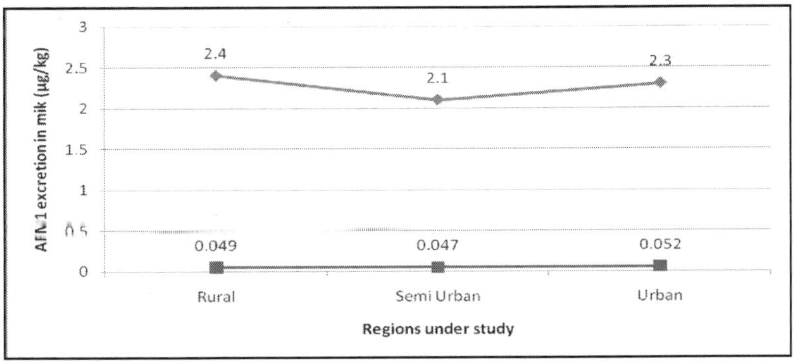


**Fig. 10:** Variations in $AFM_1$ excretion in milk (µg/day) and carry-over rate in rural, semi-urban and urban areas of cows of first lactation (after first calving) stage.

In the third lactation (calving cycle) of the cows, it was observed that the dietary intake of feed of the cows of all three localities under study increased and also there was subsequent rise in milk yield. The milk obtained from cows of rural areas had minimum $AFM_1$ content 0.049 ± 0.02µg/kg; 2.4 ± 0.48µg/day. In semi-urban areas $AFM_1$ contained 0.046 ± 0.03µg/kg; 2.1 ± 0.71µg/day. Maximum $AFM_1$ (concentration and excretion) contaminated milk was obtained from the cows of urban areas, where it was 0.051 ± 0.02µg/kg (2.3 ± 0.58 µg/day). In this lactation stage (3rd calving) also the carry-over rate of aflatoxin was the highest in the milk collected from urban areas (0.052 ± 0.009) as compared to semi-urban (0.047 ± 0.010) and rural areas (0.049 ± 0.007).

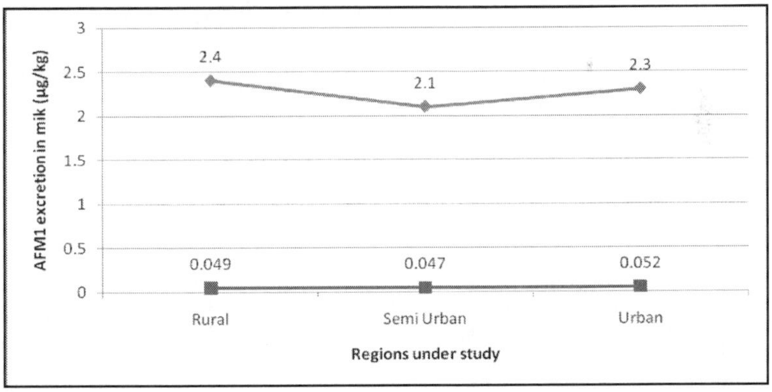


**Fig. 11:** Variations in $AFM_1$ excretion in milk (µg/day) and carry-over rate in rural, semi-urban and urban areas of cows of third lactation (after third calving) stage.

Considering the lactation/ calving cycle of the same cows (for whom first and third lactation/ calving cycle were studied), it was observed that the yield of milk increased with the increasing lactation cycle/ calving. In first calving cycle, an average of 9.8 ± 1.72 kg/day milk production was recorded in rural areas followed by 10.1 ± 1.81 kg/day in semi-urban areas and with the maximum (10.4 ± 1.53kg/ day) was recorded in the urban areas. However, in third calving cycle, the yield of milk increased to 14.1 ± 1.57 kg/day (rural areas), 13.8 ± 1.61kg/ day (semi-urban areas) and 14.3 ± 1.41 (urban areas). The level of $AFM_1$ contamination in milk was more in third lactation stage than those in first lactation/ calving cycle. The increasing trendline (in Fig - 12) showed the increase in the yield of milk of same cows from first to third calving cycle.

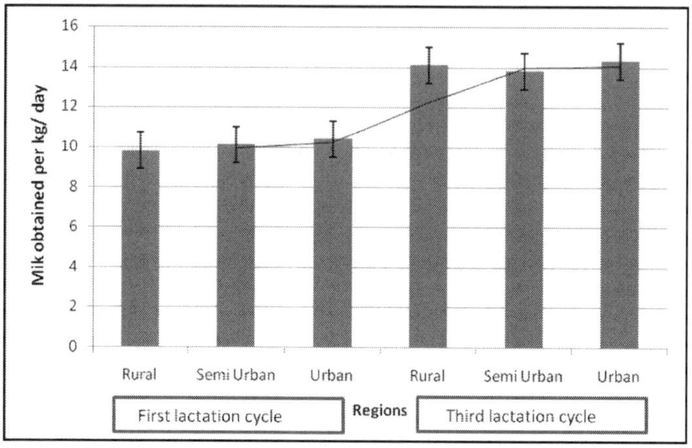


**Fig. 12:** Increase in the yield of milk with the increasing lactation/ calving cycle.

Further, the level of $AFM_1$ concentration (per kg) in milk was higher in the third calving cycle compared to first one. For the rural areas, $AFM_1$ excretion in third cycle was recorded 0.049 ± 0.02µg/kg (2.4 ± 0.48µg/day) which was followed by semi urban areas (0.046 ± 0.02µg/kg; 2.1 ± 0.71 µg/day). Maximum $AFM_1$ excretion was detected in the milk samples of urban areas (0.051 ± 0.02µg/kg; 2.3 ± 0.058µg/day). With the increased value of $AFM_1$ excretion in milk, the carry-over rate of aflatoxin in milk also increased in third calving stage compared to first one. The carry-over rate was comparatively low in semi-urban (0.047 ± 0.010) than rural areas (0.049 ± 0.007). Maximum (0.052 ± 0.009) carry-over rate was recorded in urban areas. The differences in carryover rate among them are depicted in Fig – 13.

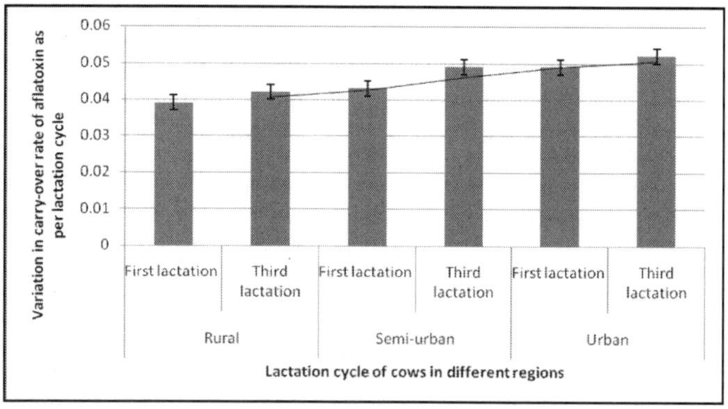


**Fig. 13:** Difference in $AFM_1$ carryover rate in first and third lactation/ calving cycle.

## C.2 Influence of Seasons on the Carryover Rate of Aflatoxin

It was desirable to monitor the influence of seasons on the carry-over rate of aflatoxins in milk samples. The variation in climatic changes in the district of

Bhagalpur and nearby areas has considerable impact on the incidence of aflatoxins and fresh and stored feeds of cows, thereby, the possibilities of their effects on the level of $AFM_1$ on milk toxin cannot be ruled out. In this locality, winter showed temperature range from 4 °C to 21°C from the month of January to March. The growth of toxigenic moulds/ spores on the feeds remained dormant at lower temperature. During the month of summer (from April to June), temperature ranged from 23°C to 45°C with low humidity. During this season high proliferations of moulds occurred. During wet season of monsoons, high temperature and high humidity favoured the excessive growth of toxigenic moulds and aflatoxin synthesis. Further, nearby areas of Bhagalpur district get water-logged during post monsoons. Wide range of temperature, humidity and their effect on the fungal growth on feeds incited us to evaluate the influence of season on carry-over rate of aflatoxin from feed to milk of cows.

Table – 16 shows the $AFB_1$ ingestion by cows in three different seasons in relation to $AFM_1$, excretion and carry-over rate. In the month of winter (January to March), the range of $AFB_1$ intake was 19.7 – 59.3µg/day, with a mean value of 38.4 ± 0.96µg per day. Whereas, $AFM_1$ concentration in milk was observed in the range of 0.016 to 0.059, with a mean value of 0.029 ± 0.006µg/ kg of milk (1.57 ± 0.09µg per day). Comparing the $AFB_1$ intake and $AFM_1$ excretion, the mean value of carry-over rate was 0.040 ± 0.001. During summer, the mean uptake of $AFB_1$ along with diet was 40.5 ±1.61µg per day and the mean $AFM_1$ concentration 0.049 ± 0.004µg/kg, (2.01 ± 0.17µg/ day). The carry-over rate was 0.054 ± 0.004. Among the seasons, the wet period of monsoons showed comparatively higher range in natural intake of $AFB_1$ and $AFM_1$ excretion which also influenced carry-over rate. Intake of $AFB_1$ was calculated in the range of 23.4 – 64.8µg per day with an average value of 42.2 ± 0.96µg/day. The range of $AFM_1$ concentration in milk was 0.036 to 0.069, with an average of 0.049 ± 0.002µg/kg. An average of 2.68 ± 0.28µg $AFM_1$ was excreted on each day during the wet seasons. The average carry-over rate during monsoon was 0.063 ± 0.008.

**Table. 16:** Influence of seasons on the carry-over rate of aflatoxin

| Seasons | Months | Range of $AFB_1$ intake (µg/day) | AFB1 intake (µg/day) (Mean) | Range of $AFM_1$ concentration in milk (µg/kg) | $AFM_1$ concentration in milk (µg/kg) (Mean) | $AFM_1$ excretion in milk (µg/day) (Mean) | Carry-over (%) |
|---|---|---|---|---|---|---|---|
| Winter | January | 19.7 - 57.1 | 37.3 ± 1.39 | 0.021 - 0.057 | 0.024 ± 0.007 | 1.50 ± 0.62 | 0.040 ± 0.007 |
| | February | 21.2 - 57.4 | 38.8 ± 1.66 | 0.016 - 0.059 | 0.027 ± 0.009 | 1.54 ± 0.89 | 0.039 ± 0.008 |
| | March | 27.6 - 59.3 | 39.1 ± 0.77 | 0.018 - 0.059 | 0.036 ± 0.009 | 1.68 ± 0.66 | 0.042 ± 0.006 |
| | **Mean** | **19.7 - 59.3** | **38.4 ± 0.96** | **0.016 - 0.059** | **0.029 ± 0.006** | **1.57 ± 0.09** | **0.040 ± 0.001** |
| Summer | April | 24.2 - 65.3 | 41.5 ± 1.68 | 0.024 - 0.061 | 0.048 ± 0.012 | 1.98 ± 0.63 | 0.052 ± 0.004 |
| | May | 36.9 - 48.6 | 38.7 ± 0.84 | 0.019 - 0.063 | 0.049 ± 0.010 | 2.11 ± 0.47 | 0.054 ± 0.005 |
| | June | 34.8 - 49.1 | 41.5 ± 1.43 | 0.024 - 0.064 | 0.050 ± 0.010 | 2.18 ± 0.77 | 0.056 ± 0.005 |
| | **Mean** | **24.2 - 65.3** | **40.5 ± 1.61** | **0.019 - 0.064** | **0.049 ± 0.004** | **2.01 ± 0.17** | **0.054 ± 0.004** |

| | | | | | | | |
|---|---|---|---|---|---|---|---|
| Monsoon | July | 28.1 - 57.2 | 42.4 ± 0.72 | 0.036 - 0.068 | 0.050 ± 0.008 | 2.47 ± 0.58 | 0.058 ± 0.002 |
| | August | 23.4 - 63.4 | 43.1 ± 1.18 | 0.040 - 0.067 | 0.051 ± 0.007 | 2.57 ± 0.34 | 0.060 ± 0.003 |
| | September | 18.6 - 64.8 | 41.2 ± 1.65 | 0.042 - 0.069 | 0.046 ± 0.006 | 3.0 ± 0.21 | 0.073 ± 0.006 |
| | **Mean** | **23.4 - 64.8** | **42.2 ± 0.96** | **0.036 - 0.069** | **0.049 ± 0.002** | **2.68 ± 0.28** | **0.063 ± 0.008** |

At p value < 0.05 for season, the mean data for carry-over rate showed significant difference between winter and monsoons. For Season X Carry-over rate, CD was 0.010 (at 5%), which clearly showed that during monsoons the mean value of carry-over was significantly higher compared to summer and winter.

Critical difference obtained through analysis of variance (ANOVA) using Microsoft excel 2013 (Microsoft, USA) and comparing data of intake of aflatoxin $B_1$ contaminated feed with respect to the carry-over rate in milk during various seasons were 0.010 ($p<0.05$). From the mean data calculated for carry-over rate of all seasons, it was evident that the value was maximum in monsoons (0.073), which, was highly significant (at $p<0.05$) compared to winters (0.040). The mean value of carry-over recorded during summer (0.054) was also significantly high to the mean value of carry-over rate of winter. However, the mean carryover rate during summer was at par with that of monsoons.

The F-value for the mean values of carry-over rate of $AFM_1$ with respect to season was also calculated using analysis of variance (ANOVA). The F value for seasons was 5.14, with the probability value of 0.001. The data thus obtained with respective degrees of freedom clearly indicated that the carry-over rate of $AFM_1$ in milk during monsoons was highly significant compared to summer and winter.

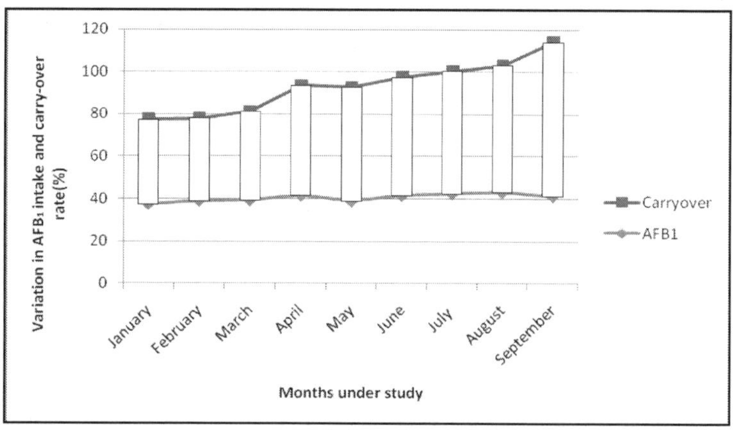


**Fig. 14:** Variation of carry-over rate of $AFM_1$ during different seasons

As evident from Fig - 14, the carry-over rate of aflatoxin in milk was independent of $AFB_1$ in the dietary intake of cows. The variation in the intake of $AFB_1$ during the ingestion of feed varied due to the variation in the spectrum of moulds with the different climatic changes. The mean value of aflatoxin $B_1$ ingestion during winter was 38.4 ± 0.96µg/day. The amount of $AFB_1$ intake increased during summer (40.5 ± 1.61µg/day) and monsoon (42.2 ± 0.96µg/day), which didn't show significant increase in value. The up-down bars in the graph showed that there was no any direct correlation with seasonal $AFB_1$ intake and carry-over rate. However, the carry-over rate showed significant differences among winter, summer and monsoon.

The maximum carry-over rate was observed during the months of monsoons i.e. in July, August, September where the peak values were 0.058, 0.060 and 0.073, respectively. In the month of August, $AFM_1$ concentration in milk was 0.051µg/kg (Fig - 15) which exceeded the EU limit. However, for rest of the months of year, the $AFM_1$ concentration in milk was found to be within the limit. The above results indicated that the $AFM_1$ contamination in raw milk was season dependent owing to the variation in the quality and type of feed given to the cows by the cattle breeders of the local areas.

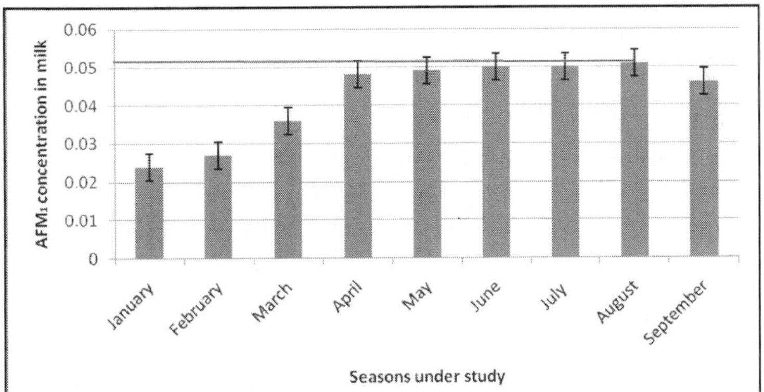


**Fig. 15:** Variations in carry-over rate of $AFM_1$ in different months/ seasons

## C.3 Influence of Age (Calving Cycles) on Carry-Over of Aflatoxin

Carry-over rate of aflatoxin from $AFB_1$ to $AFM_1$ depended on physiological state of the cows. The physiological state of individual cow might be influenced with respect to the health, nutrition (quantity and quality), habitat and age. The age of cow was one of the factors which was noticeable and thereby, an investigation in this connection was required to find out its role in carry-over of milk toxins. The lactation/ calving cycles of the cows were considered as the age factor. The carry-over rate of aflatoxin from $AFB_1$ to $AFM_1$ was studied during the milking stage in first, third and fourth lactation/ ($1^{st}$, $3^{rd}$ and $4^{th}$ calving) of the same cow. There was no marked difference in the carry over rate between first and second calving of the respective cow and so its observation was ignored (for convenience in statistical analysis). The observation of $AFB_1$ intake with the feed and corresponding yield of milk during lactation stages, the $AFM_1$ concentration in milk and its carry-over rate were recorded for each cow. These data were recorded for each cow and comparative study ($1^{st}$, $3^{rd}$ and $4^{th}$ lactation stages) of carry-over rate in the milk toxin was evaluated.

**Table 17:** Carry-over rate of milk toxin recorded in the first lactation stage (after 1st calving) of Jersey cows

| Cows | Lactation/ calving cycle of cows | $AFB_1$ intake (µg/day) (Mean) | Milk yield kg/ day (Mean) | $AFM_1$ concentration in milk (µg/kg) (Mean) | $AFM_1$ excretion in milk (µg/day) (Mean) | Carry-over rate (%) |
|---|---|---|---|---|---|---|
| C i | First | 36.1 ± 1.19 | 12.3 ± 0.87 | 0.045 ± 0.02 | 1.7 ± 0.61 | 0.041 ± 0.006 |
| C ii | First | 35.7 ± 0.82 | 13.1 ± 1.16 | 0.047 ± 0.01 | 1.5 ± 0.53 | 0.042 ± 0.007 |
| C iii | First | 34.4 ± 1.43 | 11.7 ± 1.22 | 0.042 ± 0.04 | 1.3 ± 0.12 | 0.036 ± 0.008 |
| C iv | First | 36.3 ± 0.74 | 14.3 ± 0.28 | 0.051 ± 0.03 | 1.9 ± 0.54 | 0.052 ± 0.008 |
| C v | First | 36.1 ± 0.94 | 13.5 ± 1.11 | 0.048 ± 0.01 | 1.6 ± 0.52 | 0.044 ± 0.010 |
| C vi | First | 35.1 ± 1.13 | 12.1 ± 0.81 | 0.044 ± 0.02 | 1.5 ± 0.82 | 0.042 ± 0.011 |
| C vii | First | 35.7 ± 1.28 | 13.3 ± 0.51 | 0.041 ± 0.01 | 1.4 ± 0.76 | 0.039 ± 0.009 |
| **Mean value** | | **35.6 ± 0.67** | **12.9 ± 0.91** | **0.045 ± 0.003** | **1.55 ± 0.19** | **0.004** |

During the first lactation cycle, the mean value of $AFB_1$ intake among cows was 35.6 ± 0.67µg/day (Table - 17). The yield of milk was observed in the range of 11.7 to 14.3 kg/day (Mean = 12.9 ± 0.91 kg/day). With the dietary intake of $AFB_1$, $AFM_1$ concentration in milk was observed in the mean range of 0.041 to 0.051µg/kg with an average value of 0.045 ± 0.003µg/kg (1.55 ± 0.19µg/day). Among the cows, **Civ** cows showed the maximum milk yield of 14.3 ± 0.28kg/day followed by **Cv** cow which yielded 13.5 ± 1.11kg/day and least production of milk was from cow labeled **Ciii** with an mean production of 11.7 ± 1.22kg/day. Comparing $AFM_1$ concentration in the milk of all cows, maximum was recorded in the milk of **Civ** cow (0.051 ± 0.03µg/kg) followed by **Cv** cow (0.048 ± 0.01µg/kg). Least $AFM_1$ concentration was observed in the milk of **Cvii** cow (0.041 ± 0.01µg/kg). However, the mean carry-over rate of aflatoxin $M_1$ during first lactation cycle (i.e. after first calving) was observed maximum in the milk of **Civ** cow (0.052 ± 0.008) (exceeding the EU limit), followed by **Cv** cow (0.044 ± 0.010) and the lowest in **Ciii** cow (0.036 ± 0.008). Mean carry-over rate recorded in first lactation cycle was 0.042 ± 0.004.

**Table 18:** Carry-over rate of milk toxin recorded in the third lactation stage (after 3rd calving) cycle of Jersey cows

| Cows | Lactation/ calving cycle of cows | $AFB_1$ intake (µg/day) (Mean) | Milk yield/ day (Mean) | $AFM_1$ concentration in milk (µg/kg) (Mean) | $AFM_1$ excretion in milk (µg/day) (Mean) | Carry-over rate (%) |
|---|---|---|---|---|---|---|
| C i | Third | 37.2 ± 1.49 | 15.8 ± 1.57 | 0.049 ± 0.01 | 1.7 ± 0.52 | 0.047 ± 0.006 |
| C ii | Third | 36.3 ± 1.71 | 16.4 ± 1.61 | 0.053 ± 0.03 | 1.5 ± 0.41 | 0.044 ± 0.007 |

| C iii | Third | 35.7 ± 1.43 | 14.3 ± 1.41 | 0.050 ± 0.04 | 1.5 ± 0.47 | 0.042 ± 0.008 |
|---|---|---|---|---|---|---|
| C iv | Third | 37.7 ± 1.74 | 18.4 ± 0.82 | 0.051 ± 0.01 | 2.1 ± 0.45 | 0.055 ± 0.008 |
| C v | Third | 38.5 ± 0.94 | 16.9 ± 1.41 | 0.045 ± 0.01 | 1.9 ± 0.63 | 0.052 ± 0.009 |
| C vi | Third | 37.3 ± 1.01 | 15.3 ± 1.2 | 0.046 ± 0.02 | 1.8 ± 0.71 | 0.048 ± 0.011 |
| C vii | Third | 36.2 ± 0.88 | 17.7 ± 0.95 | 0.052 ± 0.01 | 1.9 ± 0.46 | 0.049 ± 0.010 |
| **Mean value** | | **36.9 ± 0.97** | **16.4 ± 1.41** | **0.049 ± 0.002** | **1.7 ± 0.22** | **0.004** |

At p value < 0.05, for the third lactation cycle, the mean data of carry-over rate of aflatoxin $AFB_1$ to $AFM_1$ in milk showed significant differences from the carry-over rate of first lactation cycle. For statistical analysis of lactation cycle X carry-over rate, CD was 2.16 (at 5%) which clearly showed that mean value of carry-over rate in the milk obtained during third lactation cycle was significantly higher compared to that obtained during first lactation cycle.

Table - 18 shows the collected average data of $AFB_1$ ingested by the same cows during their third lactation cycle (after 3rd calving) and subsequently the data for $AFM_1$ concentration in milk (µg/kg; µg/day) and carry-over rate of toxin was recorded. The mean uptake of $AFB_1$ with the dietary intake was 36.9 ± 0.97µg/day during the third lactation cycle of same cows. It was noticeable that food intake of cows (kg/day) had increased by almost 4-5 kgs during these periods. This increase of dietary intake eventually was observed to raise the mean uptake of $AFB_1$ in third lactation cycle (or after third calving). The mean value of milk yield was 16.4 ± 1.41kg/day. The average production of milk increased as compared to first lactation cycle. The mean value of $AFM_1$ concentration and carry-over rate was 0.049 ± 0.002µg/ kg (1.7 ± 0.22µg/ day) and 0.048 ± 0.004, respectively.

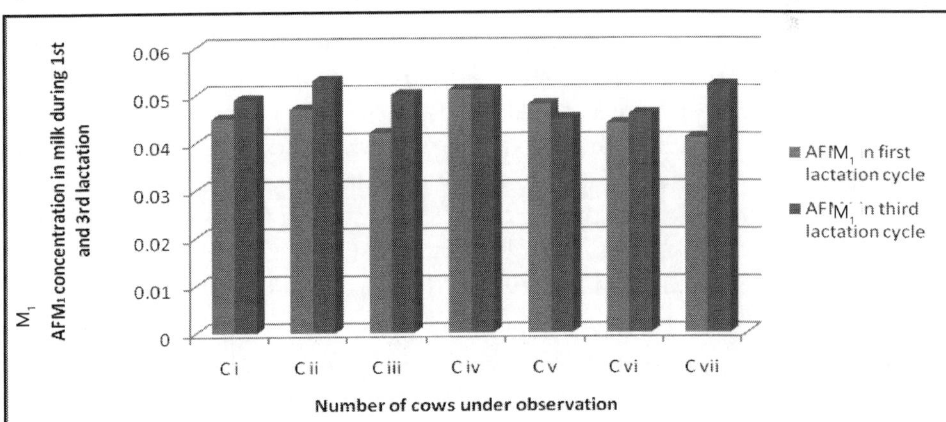


**Fig. 16:** Graph indicating the variations in $AFM_1$ concentration in milk of first and third lactation cycle (after 1st and 3rd calving)

While comparing the two lactation cycles, it was observed that mean $AFB_1$ intake increased corresponding to higher dietary intake in third lactating cycle. The $AFM_1$ concentration was observed maximum in **Cii** cow (0.053 ± 0.03µg/kg) with an average milk yield of 16.4 ± 1.61kg/day, followed by **Civ** cow (0.051 ± 0.01µg/kg) producing average milk of 18.4 ± 0.82kg/day. Lowest level of $AFM_1$ was observed in **Cv** (0.045 ± 0.01 µg/kg) with an average milk production of 16.9 ± 1.41kg/day. It is evident from the graphical figure (Fig - 16) that there was corresponding increase in the mean value of $AFM_1$ concentration in milk among the cows during third lactation cycle compared to the first.

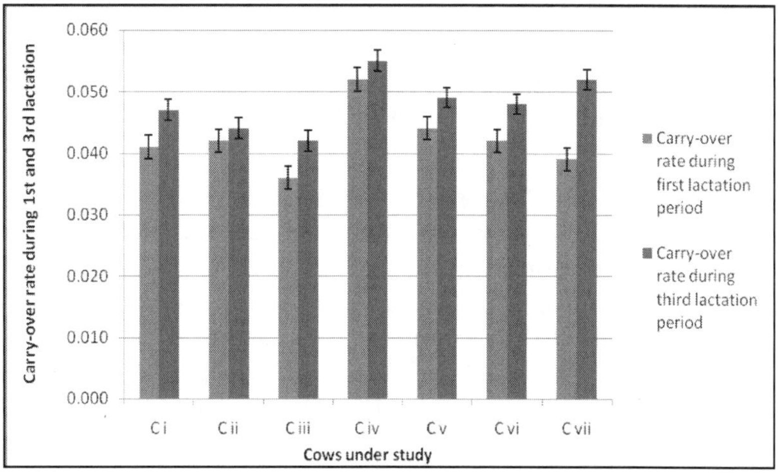


**Fig. 17:** Graph indicating the variation in carry-over of toxin in milk during first and third lactation

Variations in carry-over rate of aflatoxin in milk during first and third lactation periods were observed (Fig - 17). It was evident from the graph that there was an increase in average milk production from first lactation (12.9 ± 0.91kg/day) to third lactation (16.4 ± 1.41kg/day) and thereby, an elevation in the mean value of carry-over of aflatoxin was also observed. However, considering any of the cow as single case, no such correlation was recorded. During first lactation, the average milk production and carry-over rate was maximum in **Civ** cow (14.3 ± 0.28kg/day) followed by **Cv** cow (13.5 ± 1.11kg/day) and during third lactation maximum milk production by **Civ** cow (18.4 ± 0.82kg/day), however, carry-over rate was maximum in **Civ** cow (0.055 ± 0.008) followed by **Cv** cow (0.052 ± 0.010).

Average ingestion of $AFB_1$ by the cows during fourth lactation calving cycle and it's effect on the $AFM_1$ concentration/ excretion and carry-over rate of toxin were also monitored. The average production of milk (kg/ day) decreased to 14.3 ± 1.27kg/day in comparison to the production in third lactation stage (16.4 ± 1.41kg/day), however, dietary intake of $AFB_1$ was slightly higher in fourth lactation cycle (37.1 ± 0.67µg/day) than third lactation cycle (36.9 ± 0.97µg/day). The mean value of $AFM_1$ excretion in milk of cows during fourth lactation cycle was 0.048 ± 0.002µg/kg (1.61 ± 0.24µg/day). Comparing $AFB_1$ intake and $AFM_1$

excretion, the carry-over rate of aflatoxin in milk of the cows of fourth lactation cycle was 0.043 ± 0.005.

**Table 19:** Carry-over rate of milk toxin recorded in fourth lactation stage (after 4th calving) of Jersey cows

| Cows | Lactation/ calving cycle cows | $AFB_1$ intake (µg/day) (Mean) | Milk yield/ day (Mean) Kg ± SD | $AFM_1$ concentration in milk (µg/kg) (Mean) | $AFM_1$ excretion in milk (µg/day) (Mean) | Carry-over rate (%) |
|---|---|---|---|---|---|---|
| C i | Fourth | 36.8 ± 1.62 | 13.6 ± 1.72 | 0.047 ± 0.02 | 1.6 ± 0.58 | 0.043 ± 0.007 |
| C ii | Fourth | 37.1 ± 0.91 | 14.2 ± 1.81 | 0.049 ± 0.03 | 1.7 ± 0.62. | 0.045 ± 0.010 |
| C iii | Fourth | 36.4 ± 1.84 | 12.6 ± 1.53 | 0.045 ± 0.02 | 1.5 ± 0.56 | 0.041 ± 0.009 |
| C iv | Fourth | 38.1 ± 1.59 | 16.6 ± 0.67 | 0.052 ± 0.03 | 2 ± 0.64 | 0.052 ± 0.009 |
| C v | Fourth | 37.9 ± 1.01 | 14.3 ± 1.14 | 0.048 ± 0.02 | 1.8 ± 0.42 | 0.047 ± 0.010 |
| C vi | Fourth | 36.4 ± 1.24 | 14.1 ± 0.86 | 0.048 ± 0.01 | 1.3 ± 0.79 | 0.035 ± 0.006 |
| C vii | Fourth | 36.9 ± 1.45 | 15.3 ± 1.53 | 0.049 ± 0.01 | 1.4 ± 0.32 | 0.037 ± 0.007 |
| **Mean value** | | **37.1 ± 0.67** | **14.3 ± 1.27** | **0.048 ± 0.002** | **1.61 ± 0.24** | **0.005** |

At p value < 0.05, for the fourth lactation cycle, the mean data of carry-over rate of aflatoxin $AFB_1$ to $AFM_1$ in milk showed no significant differences in the carry-over rate of first/ third lactation cycle under observations. For statistical analysis of lactation cycle X Carry-over rate, CD was 2.16 (at 5%), which showed that mean value of carry-over rate in the milk obtained during fourth lactation cycle was non-significant compared to that obtained during first/ third lactation cycle.

The comparative study of the carry-over of milk toxin among first, third and fourth lactation cycle with respect to $AFB_1$ intake and $AFM_1$ excretion was made. The intake of $AFB_1$ through feed was 35.6 ± 0.67µg/day during first lactation cycle, which was found to increase during the third lactation cycle (36.9 ± 0.97 µg/day) and fourth lactation cycle (37.1 ± 0.67) of cows. There was increase in the diet (feed) of cows with the corresponding increase in the age of cows. For each cow, the yields of milk during those lactation cycles were quite remarkable as mean production of milk from the cows of first lactation cycle was 16.4 ± 1.41kg/day which increased to 16.4 ± 1.41kg/day during third lactation cycle, however, milk yield decreased to 14.3 ± 1.27kg/day during fourth lactation cycle. The level of $AFM_1$ excretion during those periods varied, however, showed no correlation. The average value of $AFM_1$ excretion was maximum during third lactating cycle (0.049 ± 0.002 µg/kg) followed by fourth lactating cycle (0.048 ± 0.002µg/kg), however, it was least in first lactating cycle (0.045 ± 0.003µg/kg).

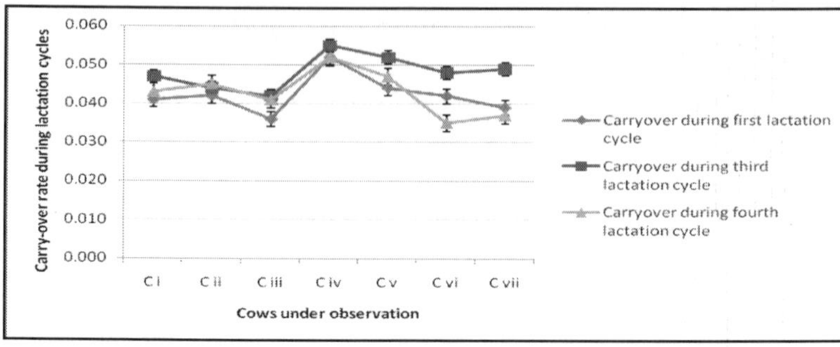


**Fig. 18:** Graphical representation of variation in carry-over rate of aflatoxin in the milk of cows during first, third and fourth lactating cycle

The carry-over rate was maximum during third lactation cycle (0.048 ± 0.004) followed by fourth lactating cycle (0.043 ± 0.005) and it was the lowest in first lactating cycle (0.042 ± 0.004). Fig – 18 showed the variations in carry-over rates of different post calving stages of cows. The excretion of $AFM_1$ (which is the product of post metabolism of $AFB_1$) is disposed through various modes from the cow. Those methods of discharging $AFM_1$ include urine, bile, faeces and milk. Hence, the physiology of cows had pronounced impact on the carry-over rate of aflatoxin from feed to milk. Variations were also observed in the mean value of milk yields and carry-over rate of each lactation cycle.

## C.4 Influence of Breeds (Individuals) on Carry-over Rate

The milk obtained from different breeds (individuals) of cows of Bhagalpur and nearby localities were considered for the observation of the carry-over rate of milk toxin. About 9 breeds of cows which included Jersey, Sahiwal, Holstein Friesein, Bachaur, Gangaitri, Gir, Harynavi, Red Sindhi and Taylor were tested for secretion of $AFM_1$ level in milk. Average intake of the quantity of foods (TMR) by those breeds were 13 kgs – 17 kgs. However, the daily milk yield showed wide variations. Some breeds (Gir, Gangaitri, Bachaur) were low milk yielding cows while Holstein Friesian, Taylor, Jersey were observed as high milk yielding cows. Table – 20 showed a comparative study of carry-over rate of aflatoxin in milk among the different breeds of cows.

**Table 20:** Variation in carry-over rate of milk toxin in different breeds of cows.

| Breeds | $AFB_1$ intake (µg/day) (Mean) | Milk yield (kg/day) (Mean) | Range of $AFM_1$ concentration in milk (µg/kg) | $AFM_1$ concentration in milk (µg/kg) (Mean) | $AFM_1$ excretion in milk (µg/day) (Mean) | Carry-over rate (%) |
|---|---|---|---|---|---|---|
| Jersey | 39.4 ± 1.39 | 12.4 ± 1.32 | 0.031 - 0.058 | 0.046 ± 0.007 | 1.60 ± 0.62 | 0.038 ± 0.004 |
| Sahiwal | 38.9 ± 1.21 | 8.7 ± 1.48 | 0.026 - 0.049 | 0.037 ± 0.009 | 1.44 ± 0.89 | 0.032 ± 0.001 |
| Holstein Friesian | 38.4 ± 1.34 | 18.1 ± 0.23 | 0.038 - 0.069 | 0.048 ± 0.009 | 2.88 ± 0.66 | 0.051 ± 0.007 |
| Bachaur | 37.8 ± 0.77 | 6.3 ± 1.18 | 0.014 - 0.047 | 0.026 ± 0.012 | 1.24 ± 0.33 | 0.027 ± 0.010 |

| Gangaitri | 38.9 ± 1.27 | 7.1 ± 1.63 | 0.018 - 0.053 | 0.031 ± 0.011 | 1.24 ± 0.47 | 0.029 ± 0.003 |
|---|---|---|---|---|---|---|
| Gir | 39.2 ± 1.31 | 4.5 ± 1.78 | 0.021 - 0.044 | 0.019 ± 0.010 | 1.28 ± 0.77 | 0.023 ± 0.011 |
| Haryanavi | 37.6 ± 1.74 | 11.4 ± 1.12 | 0.036 - 0.051 | 0.045 ± 0.002 | 1.62 ± 0.81 | 0.041 ± 0.007 |
| Red Sindhi | 38.8 ± 1.55 | 9.7 ± 0.89 | 0.030 - 0.047 | 0.047 ± 0.008 | 1.47 ± 0.54 | 0.039 ± 0.008 |
| Taylor | 38.4 ± 1.67 | 17.4 ± 1.24 | 0.032 - 0.062 | 0.051 ± 0.004 | 3.1 ± 0.71 | 0.063 ± 0.005 |

Cow breed types and the quantity of $AFM_1$ excretion were monitored during the investigation period of this study. The dietary intakes was about 3-5 kgs of maize/ wheat cake + 3-4 kgs of green grass + 6 – 8 kgs of paddy/ wheat straws mixed with maize grains. With the intake of those feeds, average $AFB_1$ intake was 38.6 ± 0.61µg/day. The range of $AFM_1$ excretion and carry-over rate in milk toxin for all breeds under these investigations were recorded.

Among the various breeds, Gir cows showed the lowest level of $AFM_1$ excretion 0.019 ± 0.010 µg/kg; 1.28 ± 0.77 µg/day where the milk yield (4.5 ± 1.78 kg/day) was also low. The Bachaur, Gangaitri, Sahiwal and Red Sindhi breeds of cows showed comparatively higher levels of $AFM_1$ excretion which were 1.24 ± 0.33 µg/ day, 1.24 ± 0.47 µg/ day, 1.44 ± 0.89 µg/ day, 1.47 ± 0.54 µg/ day, respectively. The highest 3.1 ± 0.71 µg/day level of $AFM_1$ was observed in Taylor breed of cows, the average milk yield of this breed was 17.4 ± 1.24 kg/day. The milk toxin recorded from Holstein Friesian breed of cows followed the Taylor breed cows in $AFM_1$ excretion (2.88 ± 0.66 µg/day). However, the range of $AFM_1$ concentration (0.038 - 0.069µg/kg) and milk yield (18.1 ± 0.23kg/day) of Holstein Friesian breed was comparatively higher than Taylor breed where the $AFM_1$ range was 0.032 - 0.062 µg/kg and milk yield was 17.4 ± 1.24 kg/day. In Jersey breed the range of $AFM_1$ excretion was 0.031 - 0.058 µg/kg with the mean value of 0.046 ± 0.007 µg/kg (1.60 ± 0.62 µg/day).

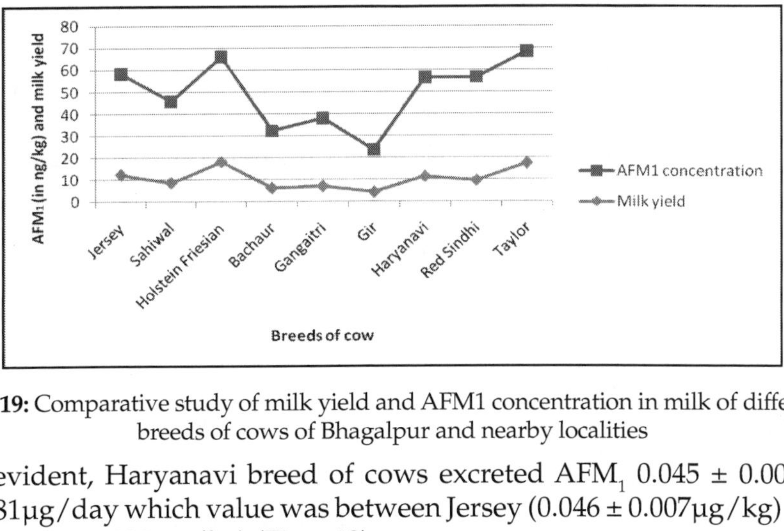


**Fig. 19:** Comparative study of milk yield and AFM1 concentration in milk of different breeds of cows of Bhagalpur and nearby localities

As evident, Haryanavi breed of cows excreted $AFM_1$ 0.045 ± 0.002µg/kg; 1.62 ± 0.81µg/day which value was between Jersey (0.046 ± 0.007µg/kg) and Red Sindhi (0.047 ± 0.008 µg/kg) (Fig – 19).

The carry-over rate of milk toxin showed a considerable variations among the different breeds of cows. The maximum (0.063 ± 0.005) carry-over rate was observed in the milk of Taylor breeds followed by Holstein Friesian (0.051 ± 0.007). Haryanavi and Jersey recorded the carry-over rate of 0.041 ± 0.007 and 0.038 ± 0.004, respectively which was lower as compared to the Taylor and Holstein Friesian. Least carry-over rate was observed in the Gir, Bachaur and Gangaitri where it was 0.023 ± 0.011, 0.027 ± 0.010 and 0.029 ± 0.003, respectively.

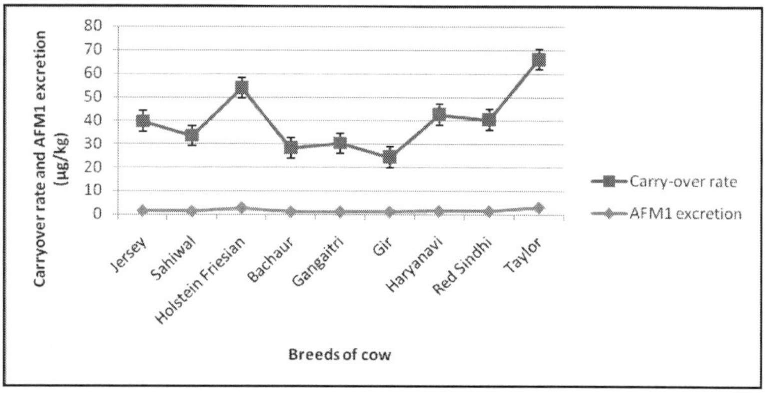


**Fig. 20:** Variations in AFM1 excretion (µg/day) and carry-over (along with standard error) among the different breeds of cows.

The mean value of $AFM_1$ concentration in the milk was determined in the unit of µg/kg for each breed of cow. Taylor breed of cows showed the maximum mean value of $AFM_1$ concentration in milk (0.051 ± 0.004µg/kg) which was slightly higher than the EU regulatory limit. However, $AFM_1$ concentration in all other breeds of cows was within the limit as set by EU. However, it has been observed that the carry-over rate was related to the milk yielding capabilities of respective cows. The carry-over rate in high milk yielding cows (Holstein Friesian, Taylor and Jersey) was comparatively higher than low yielding cows (Gir, Bachaur, Gangaitri) (Fig - 20).

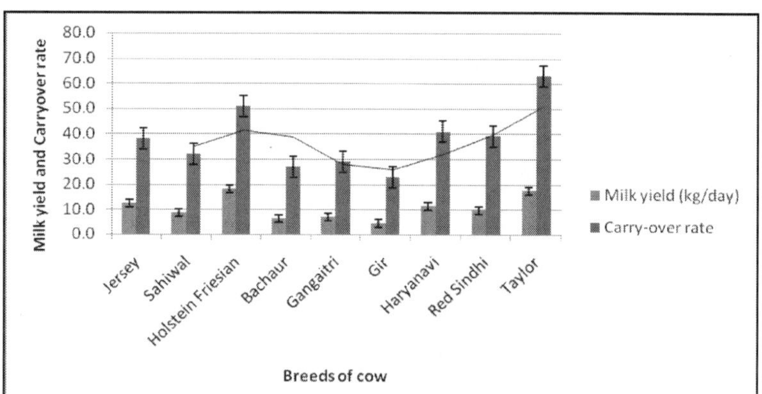


**Fig. 21:** Carry-over rate and milk yield of different breeds of cow (under study) in Bhagalpur and nearby districts.

The food intake of the cows of different breeds was in range of 13 - 22 kgs of feed per day. However, the yield of milk varied to a considerable extent. The role of individual's metabolic activities in metabolizing $AFB_1$ (with the dietary intake) into milk toxin ($AFM_1$) is a vital process. The breeds with low milk yield might have more $AFB_1$ passing through urine, bile or dung (faeces) or with less capability of $AFB_1$ conversion to milk toxin. The breed of cows with higher milk yield have more food getting metabolized into milk, thereby there are the chances of more $AFB_1$ (along with feed) getting metabolized into milk toxin ($AFM_1$). Fig – 19 and 21 showed that the higher milk yield had higher carry-over rate of $AFM_1$ concentration in milk.

## D. Levels of Aflatoxin $M_1$ in Milk Components

The carry-over rate of aflatoxin was monitored considering various perspectives such as seasonal, regional, age and breed dependant. Further, it was felt desirable to investigate the aflatoxin $M_1$ contents in different components in milk and their possible role in carry-over of aflatoxin. Milk contains four main components namely: fat, solid not fat (SNF), water and minerals (in traceable form with water). The per cent composition of fat varies from 1.5 – 6.5%, solids-not-fat (SNF) 8.1 – 9.1% and water with minerals in the range of 84.4 - 90.4%. The solids-not-fat (SNF) portion mainly consists of protein (primarily casein and lactalbumin), carbohydrates (primarily lactose). Water and minerals include water content along with calcium, phosphorus and other minerals.

The per cent wise various components of milk present in raw and processed milks is shown in Table - 21. The raw milk collected from cow breeds of Bhagalpur and nearby areas contained an average of 4.26 ± 0.01 ad 4.24 ± 0.06 per cent of solids-not-fat (i.e. lactose and protein) and 3.61 ± 0.04 per cent of fat along with 87.89 ± 0.03 per cent of water and minerals. The collected milk samples were the natural milk with no processing or additives in them. Full cream, toned, double toned and skimmed milk samples were collected from recognized dairy farms.

**Table 21:** Nutritional components in different types of milk and aflatoxin $M_1$ concentration

| Components | % in raw milk | Type of milk | $AFM_1$ concentration (µg/kg) (Mean) |
|---|---|---|---|
| Lactose | 4.26 ± 0.01 | Raw milk | 0.043 ± 0.005 |
| Protein | 4.24 ± 0.06 | | |
| Fat | 3.61 ± 0.04 | | |
| Added water and minerals | 87.89 ± 0.03 | | |
| Lactose | 4.36 ± 0.02 | Full cream | 0.044 ± 0.002 |
| Protein | 4.64 ± 0.07 | | |
| Fat | 6.09 ± 0.03 | | |
| Added water and minerals | 84.91 ± 0.02 | | |

<table>
<tr><td>Lactose</td><td>4.38 ±0.01</td><td rowspan="4">Toned milk</td><td rowspan="4">0.041 ± 0.006</td></tr>
<tr><td>Protein</td><td>4.12 ±0.05</td></tr>
<tr><td>Fat</td><td>3.06 ± 0.05</td></tr>
<tr><td>Added water and minerals</td><td>88.44 ±0.07</td></tr>
<tr><td>Lactose</td><td>4.31 ±0.02</td><td rowspan="4">Double toned</td><td rowspan="4">0.038 ± 0.001</td></tr>
<tr><td>Protein</td><td>4.08 ± 0.03</td></tr>
<tr><td>Fat</td><td>1.57 ± 0.02</td></tr>
<tr><td>Added water and minerals</td><td>89.94 ± 0.07</td></tr>
<tr><td>Lactose</td><td>4.47 ± 0.03</td><td rowspan="4">Skimmed milk</td><td rowspan="4">0.014 ± 0.011</td></tr>
<tr><td>Protein</td><td>4.23 ± 0.02</td></tr>
<tr><td>Fat</td><td>0.68 ± 0.03</td></tr>
<tr><td>Added water and minerals</td><td>90.62 ± 0.08</td></tr>
</table>

Full cream milk was processed milk prepared by standardizing with addition of extra fats or mixing cow milk with buffalo milk so as to maintain a level of fats and SNFs. An average value of SNFs were 4.36 ± 0.02 (Lactose) and 4.64 ± 0.07 (Protein). Fat was present with a mean value of 6.01 ± 0.03 per cent. Water with minerals accounted 84.91 ± 0.02 per cent of total constituents. The SNFs in toned, double toned and skimmed milk were nearly similar, however, the ratio of fat was found to be remarkably different. In toned milk (also called single toned milk) is prepared by adding skimmed milk powder and water to raw milk, the fat ratio was 3.06 ± 0.05 per cent of the milk. While in double toned (prepared by adding skimmed milk powder with water to raw milk), fat per cent was approximately 1.57 ± 0.02 of the complete milk. Skimmed milk had the least per cent (0.68 ± 0.03) of fat.

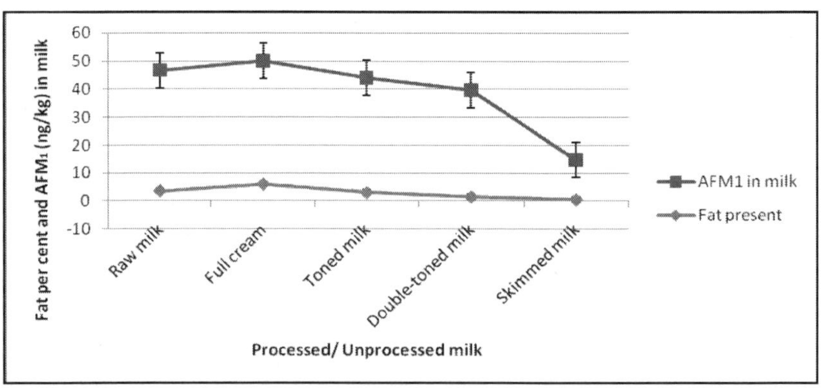


**Fig. 22:** Graphical representation of the aflatoxin variation with the per cent fat present in various processed/ unprocessed milk.

Fig – 22 depicts the graphical representation showing variations in fat per cent of the raw milk, full cream, toned, double-toned and skimmed milk and the corresponding variations in $AFM_1$ concentrations (in different processed/

unprocessed milk). At 3.61 % of fat in raw milk, mean value of $AFM_1$ present was 0.043 ± 0.005µg/kg. However, toned milk, double-toned and skimmed milk showed reduction in the mean value of $AFM_1$ 0.041 ± 0.006, 0.038 ± 0.001, 0.014 ± 0.011µg/kg, respectively, with their corresponding decrease in fat concentration in those milk. Full-cream milk showed high fat per cent (6.01 ± 0.03) compared to other types of milk, and also $AFM_1$ value 0.044 ± 0.002µg/kg, which, however, was within the EU limit. This variation can be understood with the fact that extra fat added to the raw milk was saturated processed fat, which was mixed in fixed proportion in order to maintain the quality of milk.

Unlike the types of milk, the fat constituents of dairy products showed no relation with the $AFM_1$ concentration in milk (Fig - 23). The fat concentration of butter was maximum (80%) among all the dairy products studied, however, the $AFM_1$ concentration was 0.213 ± 0.05µg/kg. Similarly, fat concentration of khoya was 36.9 and $AFM_1$ concentration varied from 0.234 µg/kg to 0.624 µg/kg.

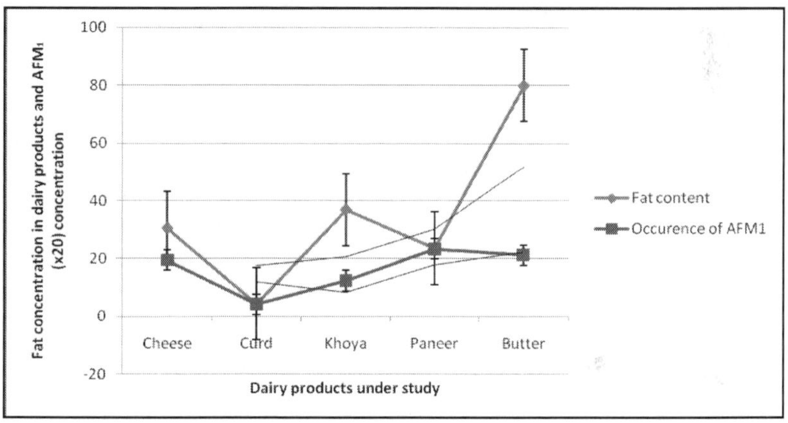


**Fig. 23:** Graphical representation of dairy products showing correlations with fat and AFM1 concentration

## E. Control Strategies to Minimize Aflatoxin in Milk

Aflatoxins in cattle feed is inevitable in Indian climatic conditions and toxins if present in cattle feed ($AFB_1$), it would get carried over to the milk ($AFM_1$). Thus two main checkpoints can be made for developing control strategies:- a) controlling aflatoxin in feeds, which needs to be checked during selection of feed, its storage and processing of feeds. B) controlling aflatoxins in milk before it reaches to consumers.

### E.1 Treatment of Cattle Feed

The primary approach for control of aflatoxin contamination can be made through preventive measures.

(i) One of the possible approaches can be made by applying effective integrated aflatoxin management systems (Preharvest, harvest, transport, storage and processing systems) based on HACCP approaches.

(ii) **Incorporation of more fresh feeds in dietary intake of cows:** Practices such as dietary intake of fresh feeds like green grasses etc. can be given to the cows (Table - 7). It was observed that fresh cattle feeds/ green feeds showed least aflatoxin contamination (Fig - 24). The mean $AFB_1$ in the fresh feeds were observed 2.06µg/kg, with 31% of the total sample beyond EU limit. However, commercial and household feeds showed large variations with regard to aflatoxin contamination.

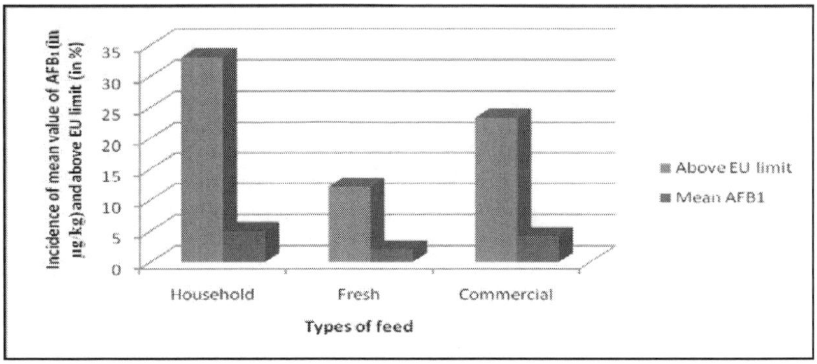


**Fig. 24:** Graphical representation of comparative incidence of $AFB_1$ (mean value and EU limit)

(iii) **Use of plant extracts, commercial phenol, volatile organic compounds:** The extracts of wild plants are known to show inhibitory effect on the growth and aflatoxin production. This concept was tried on the cattle feeds to observe the inhibition of aflatoxin, if any. The reduction per cent observed has been summarized in the Table – 22.

**Table 22:** Effect of plant extracts/ commercial phenolics/ volatile organic compounds on mixed total ration (MTR) of cattle and subsequent reduction in $AFB_1$ production.

| Plant extracts/ commercial phenol/ volatile organic compounds | Mean value of $AFB_1$ (µg/kg) (Control) | Mean reduction in $AFB_1$ | % reduction in $AFB_1$ content |
|---|---|---|---|
| *Azadirachta indica A. Juss* | 4.3 ± 0.94 | 2.05 ± 0.78 | 52.4 |
| *Euphorbia hirta L.* | 3.9 ± 1.67 | 2.06 ± 0.54 | 36.8 |
| *Ocimum sanctum L.* | 4.1 ± 1.14 | 3.07 ± 0.72 | 25.1 |
| *Ricinus communis L.* | 2.8 ± 1.09 | 2.13 ± 0.66 | 23.7 |
| *Thuja orientalis L.* | 3.4 ± 0.68 | 2.39 ± 0.79 | 29.5 |
| Tannic acid | 5.1 ± 1.29 | 4.05 ± 0.56 | 20.4 |
| Acetic acid | 4.7 ± 0.37 | 3.91 ± 0.43 | 83.1 |
| Acetone | 3.8 ± 1.21 | 2.94 ± 0.85 | 22.5 |
| Formaldehyde | 4.02 ± 1.53 | 2.48 ± 0.36 | 38.2 |
| Propionic acid | 2.9 ± 1.72 | 1.76 ± 0.61 | 39.1 |

The inhibition per cent through different treatments (with plant extracts, phenolics and volatile organic compounds) was observed in the range of 20-83% of the $AFB_1$ contents in mixed total ration (MTR) of cattle. The organic volatile compound (acetic acid) showed the maximum reduction (83.1%) in aflatoxin contamination. Among the plant extracts, *Azadirachta indiaca* A. Juss showed the maximum per cent reduction (52.4) in $AFB_1$, followed by Propionic acid (39.1%). Formaldehyde resulted in 38.2% inhibition of aflatoxin synthesis in the composite cattle feed substrates. In case of treatment with the herbal extracts of *Euphorbia hirta* L., *Thuja orientalis* L., *Ocimum sanctum* L. and *Ricinus communis* L., the inhibition per cent observed were 36.8, 29.5, 25.1 and 23.7, respectively. Commercial phenolics (Tannic acid) showed the least reduction (20.4%) of aflatoxin contents.

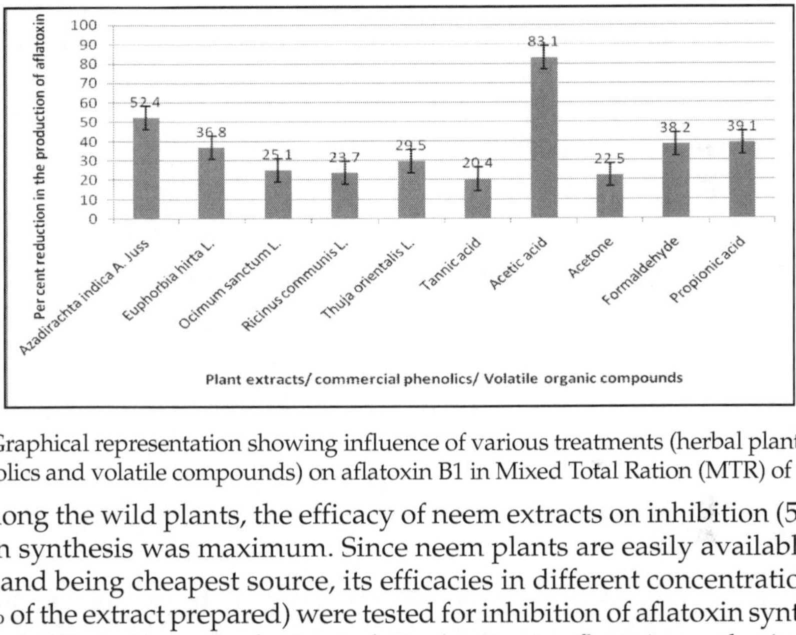


**Fig. 25:** Graphical representation showing influence of various treatments (herbal plant extracts, phenolics and volatile compounds) on aflatoxin B1 in Mixed Total Ration (MTR) of cattle.

Among the wild plants, the efficacy of neem extracts on inhibition (52.4%) of aflatoxin synthesis was maximum. Since neem plants are easily available in this locality and being cheapest source, its efficacies in different concentrations (10% and 50% of the extract prepared) were tested for inhibition of aflatoxin synthesis on cattle feed. Effect of neem leaf extracts for reduction in aflatoxin synthesis on cattle feed ingredients (main dietary component of cows) were evaluated. Remarkable effects of neem extracts were observed for reduction in aflatoxin synthesis on various cattle feed components. Reduction in the synthesis of aflatoxin $B_1$ was observed in the range of 4.3 to 47.2% (Table - 23).

**Table 23:** Effect of different concentrations of neem extract in the reduction of aflatoxin $B_1$ synthesis on cattle feeds.

| Substrates | $AFB_1$ (µg/kg) (mean) | Treatment with neem extract for 48 hours | Range of reduction in $AFB_1$ (µg/kg) | Reduction in $AFB_1$ (µg/kg) (mean) | Range of % reduction in $AFB_1$ | % Reduction in $AFB_1$ |
|---|---|---|---|---|---|---|
| Wheat bran | 3.6 ± 1.24 | 10% | 2.8 - 3.7 | 3.4 ± 0.24 | 1% - 17% | 5.02 |
| | | 50% | 1.8 - 2.4 | 2.08 ± 0.36 | 33.3% - 47.2% | 42.3 |

| Paddy straw | 3.9 ± 1.44 | 10% | 2.9 - 4.1 | 3.6 ± 0.41 | 0.5 - 19% | 7.03 |
|---|---|---|---|---|---|---|
| | | 50% | 1.7 - 2.8 | 2.1 ± 0.22 | 28% - 71% | 47.2 |
| Maize grains | 2.43 ± 0.31 | 10% | 1.4 - 2.7 | 2.2 ± 0.17 | 2% - 12.7% | 9.5 |
| | | 50% | 0.8 - 1.8 | 1.3 ± 0.28 | 25% - 66.6% | 46.5 |
| Crushed maize | 4.6 ± 0.37 | 10% | 3.5 - 4.3 | 4 ± 0.34 | 6.5% - 23.9 | 13 |
| | | 50% | 1.2 - 3.1 | 2.03 ± 0.61 | 38.8% - 57.9% | 41.6 |
| Paddy husk | 4.7 ± 0.62 | 10% | 3.9 - 4.7 | 4.5 ± 0.83 | 1% - 17.02% | 4.3 |
| | | 50% | 2.1 - 3.6 | 2.9 ± 0.66 | 23.4% - 55.3% | 39.3 |

Cattle feeds were treated with crude extracts of neem for 48 hours. $AFB_1$ quantification of pre and post treated cattle feeds were made. The substrates used (for treatment) were the typical cattle feeds mostly fed to cattle at Bhagalpur and nearby districts. Maximum reduction (47.2%) was observed in the paddy straw when treated with 50% crude neem extract followed by maize grains (46.5%), however, least reduction (39.3%) was observed in the paddy husk.

(iv) **Use of light sources on the reduction of aflatoxin synthesis in maize grains:**

**Table 24:** Effect of different kinds of light on the inhibition of $AFB_1$ synthesis on maize grain (important ingredient of cattle feed)

| **Substrates** | **$AFB_1$ (µg/kg) (mean)** | **Type of lights** | **Reduction in $AFB_1$ (µg/kg) (mean)** | **% reduction in $AFB_1$** |
|---|---|---|---|---|
| Maize grains | 4.2 ± 0.72 | Sunlight | 3.69 ± 0.64 | 12 |
| Maize grains | 3.8 ± 1.23 | Tubelight | 3.72 ± 0.42 | 2 |
| Maize grains | 3.6 ± 0.34 | Bulb light | 3.45 ± 0.67 | 4 |
| Maize grains | 4.08 ± 0.89 | UV light | 3.14 ± 0.38 | 23 |

The effects of different of lights were observed on the production of $AFB_1$ in maize grains (Table - 24). Tubelight showed the minimum reduction (2%), followed by bulb light which comparatively showed greater reduction (4%) of the $AFB_1$ in maize grains. UV light showed the maximum reduction (23%) of aflatoxin $B_1$ in maize. Sun dried maize grains showed 12% reduction in aflatoxin $B_1$ contents.

## E.2 Treatment of Milk

Strategic control of aflatoxin $M_1$ in milk may involve utilization of certain absorbents in the diet of cattle, heating/ ultra heating/ pasteurization of milk or using fat free milk.

**(i) Use of Activated Carbon to reduce the aflatoxin carry-over in milk:**

The test cows in first week were not fed with any absorbent, however, just the usual diet was given. In the second week, activated carbon (2%) as absorbent was given to the cows mixed with the normal dietary uptake. The presence of activated carbon rendered black colour to the meal of the cattle. It was observed that the amounts of feed ingested by cows were not affected by the addition of activated carbon.

**Table 25:** Reduction in the carry-over rate of aflatoxin $B_1$ to $M_1$ with the intake of activated carbon by the cows.

| Weeks | Cows | Adsorbent in feed | $AFB_1$ intake (µg/day) (mean) | Milk yield (kg/day) (mean) | $AFM_1$ concentration (µg/kg) (mean) | $AFM_1$ excretion (µg/day) (mean) | Carry-over rate (%) | Reduction in carry-over rate (%) |
|---|---|---|---|---|---|---|---|---|
| Week 1 | Cow 1 | None | 35.6 ± 0.85 | 12.9 ± 0.86 | 0.043 ± 0.01 | 1.5 ± 0.53 | 0.042 ± 0.007 | NA |
| | Cow 2 | None | 34.3 ± 1.61 | 11.2 ± 1.34 | 0.042 ± 0.04 | 1.1 ± 0.12 | 0.036 ± 0.008 | NA |
| | Cow 3 | None | 36.7 ± 1.22 | 15.6 ± 0.18 | 0.051 ± 0.03 | 1.9 ± 0.54 | 0.052 ± 0.008 | NA |
| | Cow 4 | None | 37.2 ± 0.58 | 14.1 ± 1.17 | 0.048 ± 0.01 | 1.7 ± 0.52 | 0.044 ± 0.010 | NA |
| | Cow 5 | None | 32.8 ± 1.54 | 10.6 ± 1.62 | 0.036 ± 0.02 | 1.3 ± 0.82 | 0.042 ± 0.011 | NA |
| Week 2 | Cow 1 | Activated carbon | 36.2 ± 0.82 | 12.6 ± 1.36 | 0.047 ± 0.03 | 1.6 ± 0.36 | 0.027 ± 0.003 | 35.7 |
| | Cow 2 | Activated carbon | 35.5 ± 1.43 | 12.1 ± 1.22 | 0.045 ± 0.01 | 1.1 ± 0.27 | 0.020 ± 0.004 | 44.4 |
| | Cow 3 | Activated carbon | 34.2 ± 0.74 | 15.2 ± 0.26 | 0.050 ± 0.06 | 1.7 ± 0.42 | 0.030 ± 0.008 | 42.3 |
| | Cow 4 | Activated carbon | 35.7 ± 0.94 | 13.9 ± 1.11 | 0.044 ± 0.02 | 1.3 ± 0.48 | 0.037 ± 0.012 | 15.9 |
| | Cow 5 | Activated carbon | 34.7 ± 1.28 | 10.1 ± 0.81 | 0.037 ± 0.05 | 1.5 ± 0.62 | 0.031 ± 0.009 | 26.2 |

For control set of experiments, five test cows were selected and in the first week they were fed with normal feed and aflatoxin $B_1$ intake, $M_1$ excretion and carry-over rate were observed. Table – 25 showed the remarkable reduction in carryover rate of aflatoxin with the intake of activated carbon (2%) along with cattle meal. The activated carbon was fed to the same cows in second week. Reduction in carryover rate was observed in the range of 15.9 to 44.4 per cent. This was done to maintain the standard physiology of cows for the experimental purposes. **Cow 4** showed the lowest reduction (15.9%) in carryover, however, **Cow 2** showed maximum reduction (44.4%) in carryover rate followed by **Cow 3** (42.3%).

### (ii) Heat treatment of milk

The raw milk procured from cattle breeders were subjected to various heating treatments. The experiment was carried out to observe the effect of mild heating, pasteurization, high and ultra high heating treatments on $AFM_1$ concentration of milk. Table – 26 shows the outcome of the reduction in $AFM_1$ concentration of raw milk which was partly divided into various fixed volumes and were subjected to evaluate the heating effects.

**Table 26:** Effect of heating conditions on $AFM_1$ concentration of milk

| Heat conditions | Raw milk (AFM1 µg/kg) (mean) | Post treatment (mean) | % Reduction |
|---|---|---|---|
| 61 C for 15 mins | 0.041 ± 0.005 | 0.039 ± 0.002 | 4.88% |
| 61 C for 30 mins | 0.041 ± 0.005 | 0.039 ± 0.003 | 4.86% |
| Pasteurization (71.6 C for 15 sec) | 0.041 ± 0.005 | 0.038 ± 0.003 | 7.30% |
| 75 C for 15 mins | 0.041 ± 0.005 | 0.035 ± 0.001 | 14.61% |
| 75 C for 30 mins | 0.041 ± 0.005 | 0.035 ± 0.004 | 14.57% |
| 100 C for 15 mins | 0.041 ± 0.005 | 0.033 ± 0.007 | 19.51% |
| 100 C for 30 mins | 0.041 ± 0.005 | 0.032 ± 0.002 | 21.95% |
| 121 C for 20 mins | 0.041 ± 0.005 | 0.026 ± 0.006 | 36.58% |
| Ultra heating (140 C for 3 sec) | 0.041 ± 0.005 | 0.024 ± 0.009 | 41.46% |

Ultra-heating (UHT) performed at 140 C for 3 seconds showed the maximum reduction (41.46%) of $AFM_1$ content of milk. The $AFM_1$ content in raw milk which was subjected to different heating conditions was 0.041µg/kg and at UHT, the level of aflatoxin $M_1$ content was 0.024 ± 0.009µg/kg. The sudden high temperature is known to kill various spores of bacteria and fungus as well. After UHT, temperature treatment at 121°C for 20 minutes the level of $AFM_1$ content was 0.026 ± 0.006µg/kg. As obvious from the proceeding trendline of the graph (Fig - 26), the time duration of heating plays an important role than only temperature itself. The temperature rise between 75°C to 100°C showed no reduction, however, maintaining the temperature of 100°C for 30 mints led the reduction from 0.033 ± 0.007µg/kg to 0.031 ± 0.002µg/kg.

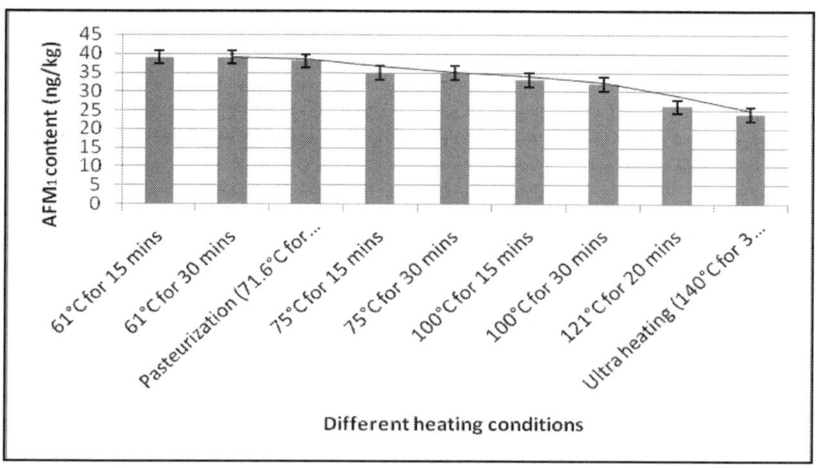


**Fig 26:** Graphical representation of different heating conditions affecting the $AFM_1$ content of the milk.

CHAPTER 4

# Discussion

## A. Qualitative and Quantitative Estimations of Aflatoxins from Cattle Feed, Milk and Milk Product

### A.1 Aflatoxin in Cattle Feed

Mycotoxins, secondary metabolites of fungi, contaminate food and feed and can cause toxic effects in cattle and human beings (Williams, 2011; Gnonlonfin *et al.*, 2013; Wu *et al.*, 2014; Hoffmann *et al.*, 2015; Obonyo and Solano, 2018). According to an estimate of FAO and WHO, about 25% of the world's crops (maize, rice, other cereals, nuts, cattle feeds etc.) are contaminated by moulds and mycotoxins (Wu *et al.*, 2007; Pandya and Arade, 2016; Lee and Ruy, 2017). Aflatoxin synthesized by *Aspergillus flavus, A. parasiticus* and *A. nomius* (Kurtzman *et al.*, 1987) is most potent human carcinogen and it is being classified as Class I human carcinogen (IARC, 2002). It is also mutagenic, teratogenic and immuno-suppressive. In subtropical countries like India the incidence of aflatoxigenic fungi remain quite high due to favourable agroclimatic conditions. Food/ feed safety is a matter of high concern during the present population growth. *A. flavus* infestation and aflatoxin synthesis can occur at any stage of crop production throughout the food chain. Several factors are known to influence aflatoxin synthesis such as presence of toxigenic inoculum, host genotype, insect activities, cultural practices, agro-climatic conditions prevailing during preharvest, harvest and storage conditions (Bilgrami *et al.*, 1991; Bilgrami and Choudhary, 1997; Choudhary and Kumari, 2010; Pleadin *et al.*, 2015; Kumari, 2018). However, in any finished animal feed, contaminated ingredients may cause contamination of the entire feed lot. When such contaminated feedstuffs are consumed by cattle, it may cause liver toxicity, mutation, alteration in metabolism, decreased disease resistance and reduced milk production (Sinha and Bhatnagar, 1997; Magan and Olsen, 2004). In the liver of cattle, $AFB_1$ is biotransformed into its hydroxylated derivatives ($AFM_1$) and from there it is transferred into the milk. There are several reports which confirmed that the levels of aflatoxin $M_1$ in milk was directly correlated to the dietary intake of aflatoxin $B_1$ in cattle feed (Prandini *et al.*, 2009; Mozafari *et al.*, 2017). Since milk is the complete food and thereby, it is being prescribed to infants, children and old aged people (Bahrami *et al.*, 2016; Costamagna *et al.*, 2019). However, those people in turn become more susceptible to the adverse effects of milk toxin ($AFM_1$) as they have comparatively low immunity. Due to the genotoxic nature of aflatoxin $M_1$, it has been categorised as class 2 B human carcinogens (IARC, 2002). Considering its high human health risk, several countries have imposed stringent regulations. Accordingly, European commission (EU) has set a maximum limit of 0.05μg/kg and 20 μg/kg for aflatoxin $B_1$ and for total aflatoxins (aflatoxin $B_1$, $B_2$, $G_1$ and $G_2$), respectively.

Cattle rearing is one of the major sources of income in rural as well as semi-urban areas of Bihar. Various agricultural produce such as maize, wheat, paddy (grains, husk or straw) and green grasses are the main dietary food of cattle. Natural incidence of mycotoxins especially aflatoxins is considerably high in Bihar due to outdated agriculture and storage practices, unseasonal rains, prevailing high temperature and relative humidity and also because of socio-economic backwardness (Bilgrami, 1990). In addition to those conditions, flood (river of Ganga, Kosi and their tributaries) is the regular feature of this locality (Bilgrami, 1990; Bilgrami and Choudhary, 1997). Thus the prevailing situations lead to excessive moistening of the grains resulting in intense mould growth and mycotoxin synthesis (Bilgrami *et al.*, 1990; Choudhary and Kumari, 2014). Previous studies from our laboratory have revealed that in Bihar no edible commodities are absolutely safe from the attack of toxigenic moulds and/ or aflatoxin/ mycotoxin contamination (Sinha, 1983; Sinha and Sinha, 1990; Bilgrami and Choudhary, 1998; Choudhary and Kumari, 2010). However, till date there was no comprehensive research on the occurrence of aflatoxin in different types of cattle feeds of this locality.

In the present investigation aflatoxin incidence on various types of cattle feeds of Bhagalpur and surrounding areas was evaluated. Influence of seasons on incidence of aflatoxin is necessary to be monitored for proper management of this toxin. In this locality cattle breeders mostly utilize three types of cattle feeds, which are commercial feed (purchased from market), household storage feed (feedstock stacked in farmyard) and fresh fodder (freshly harvested feeds). Samples of different types of cattle feeds were collected in different seasons for monitoring of $AFB_1$ incidence.

Eight genera of moulds (*Aspergillus, Fusarium, Penicillium, Rhizopus, Alternaria, Curvularia, Cladosporium* and *Mucor* spp) were isolated from cattle feed samples. The fungal spectrum varied in different seasons with the change in the climatic conditions. *A. flavus* incidence was the highest (87%) in wet seasons followed by dry (76%) and cold seasons (19%).

A total of 1130 cattle feed samples collected from different localities of the district were analysed for $AFB_1$. Among them 66.6% (753 samples) were found contaminated with $AFB_1$. High (5.02 ± 2.46μg/kg) concentration of $AFB_1$ was observed in household cattle feed samples. The amount of toxin was significantly high ($p<0.05\%$) as compared to the samples of commercial and fresh feeds. Approximately 33% of the household cattle samples had aflatoxin $B_1$ level exceeding the European Union (EU) limit. Considering different types of samples and the different seasons together, it was observed that aflatoxin $B_1$ level was maximum (mean 7.79 ± 2.0µg/kg) in monsoons of cattle feed samples, which was followed by commercial feed (5.17 ± 0.75µg/kg). It was evident from the observations that the freshly harvested feedstuffs were comparatively safe for consumption as 83-95% of the samples had aflatoxin level below the EU limit (0.05µg/kg).

During the present crisis of climatic changes, monitoring of seasonal assessment of aflatoxin $B_1$ level in different types of cattle feeds can be an important indicator for accessing aflatoxin risk. Interactions between seasons and cattle feed types in relation to aflatoxin contamination have been observed in previous studies (Wu *et al.*, 2011; Bryden, 2012; Ruscito *et al.*, 2016; Ismail *et al.*, 2017; Obonyo and Solano, 2018). In an investigation made in Bihar during 2006 – 2010, it was found that the climatic conditions correlated well with the incidence of aflatoxin in field crops (Choudhary and Kumari, 2014). Per cent viable conidia of toxigenic *A. flavus* in wet months (monsoons) were comparatively higher than in winters or summers. In this area the high temperature, % RH and outdated storage system prevailed, which provided an ideal condition for *A. flavus* infection and aflatoxin production. With the change of seasons, the incidence of fungal community and co-inhabiting mycoflora varied, possibilities of their synergistic or antagonistic effect on *A. flavus* growth cannot be ruled out (Choudhary, 1992; Choudhary and Sinha, 1993; Sinha and Choudhary, 2008).

Mean aflatoxin $B_1$ content in the samples of commercial centres had 4.19 ± 1.05 µg/kg and the range of toxin varied from 0.85µg/kg to 7.56µg/kg. 23.3 % of commercial feed samples had the toxin above the acceptable limit (0.05µg/kg) of European Union. In commercial feeds the risk of aflatoxin was high as because maize was used as the major ingredients of cattle feed (Pleadin *et al.*, 2015; Omeiza, 2019). Maize grains contain high nutritional value and also it has massive cultivation in Bihar. In this state maize is most important staple crops, being consumed as food and feed in different ways (Choudhary and Kumari, 2014). It's cultivation is made throughout the year (summer, monsoon and winter), which covers an area of 0.6 million hectares, the yearly production being 2.0 million tonnes. The harvested crops are mostly stored for future consumption as food and feedstuffs, however, the storage condition of this locality is quite poor, traditional and unhealthy. If contamination of an ingredient can occur at any stage of crop development, it may cause contamination of the entire feed lot. Farmers mostly stacked the feeds in open places in farmyard, in which later were used before those stacked earlier. Thus the earlier stacked feeds were left undisturbed throughout the year till being utilized for cattle consumption (Choudhary *et al.*, 2020). Poor and unhealthy management of drying of feeds were also observed (especially in household storage of cattle feeds). Unseasonal rain was the recurrent feature of this terrain, which resulted high moistening of the feed and thereby, providing congenial conditions for *A. flavus* infestation and aflatoxin synthesis. Freshly harvested feeds contained least amount of aflatoxin while considering the three sources of feeds. Chances of aflatoxin poisoning in cattle can be minimized through feeding them fresh fodder. It is evident from the findings that fresh feed was comparatively safe for the consumption, however, even in wet seasons maximum (83%) samples were within the limit of acceptance.

Aflatoxin contamination in cattle feed is markedly effected by seasonal variations of abiotic factors. In all the three localities under observations and also considering the types of cattle feeds, wet period showed significantly high levels ($p<0.05$) of aflatoxin contamination. Mean aflatoxin level in summer was 3.53µg/kg, however, in winters it was 2.55µg/kg.

**Aflatoxin $B_1$ Contamination in Cattle Feed of Different Localities**

In all the seasons, the cattle feed samples of Naugachia had the maximum ($4.2 \pm 1.56$ µg/kg) levels of aflatoxins followed by Bhagalpur ($3.7 \pm 1.45$ µg/kg). During monsoons the cattle feed of Naugachia contained high (11.14µg/kg) levels of aflatoxin $B_1$. In this areas, flood is the recurrent feature where maize (a major ingredients of cattle feed) is harvested mostly during late August/ early September by that time crops get submerged with flood water (Sinha, 1987). Farmers have no option but to harvest the crops before full maturity and thereby, kernels contained high moisture contents. Further processing (peeling, shelling and drying) of the crops are made on nearby National Highway. Frequent rains result in late drying of kernels. Such situations provided an ideal situation for *A. flavus* contamination and aflatoxin synthesis. Those contaminated maize kernels when mixed with the cattle feed, resulted in contamination of entire feed lots.

It is obvious that aflatoxin is an inevitable contaminants produced by *Aspergillus* group of fungi. The present investigation revealed that aflatoxin $B_1$ remained present in all types of feedstuffs of these localities. *Aspergillus flavus* was most prevalent fungus especially during monsoons and summers. The ($AFB_1$) level was comparatively high in the household feeds. Samples collected from commercial feeds also showed the high incidence of aflatoxin $B_1$ (23.3% above EU limit). It is thereby, inferred that fresh feeds were safer for consumption. With respect to seasons, in monsoons there was the highest incidence of aflatoxin contamination due to prevailing conducive environmental conditions for *A. flavus* growth and aflatoxin synthesis. Maize (a major ingredient of cattle feed) is harvested during monsoons/ onset of floods, which resulted in excessive moistening of the kernels and thereby, high incidence of *A. flavus* and aflatoxins contamination.

## A.2 Aflatoxin in Milk and Milk Products

If the lactating cattle are fed with $AFB_1$ contaminated feed then there are all possible chances of excreted milk being contaminated with $AFM_1$. (Paulin *et al.*,

2011; Aslam, 2015; Krstovic *et al.*, 2018; Choudhary *et al.*, 2020). The contamination of aflatoxin $M_1$ also occurs when the moulds synthesizing aflatoxin pass to the milk and produce aflatoxin during transport, process and storage phases after milking (Celik *et al.*, 2005). Aflatoxin $M_1$ is the monohydroxy derivative of $AFB_1$, produced after metabolization in liver following consumption of contaminated feed by lactating cows/ cattle. After ingestion of contaminated feed, $AFM_1$ can be detected in cow's milk (with the percentage of 1-6% of $AFB_1$) from few hours to two days (Gurbay *et al.*, 2006). Any dairy product prepared from $AFM_1$ contaminated milk will in turn contain aflatoxin and thereby, it would be unsafe for human consumption (Tahoun *et al.*, 2017). Dairy products are also one of the most important exposure factors through diet for $AFM_1$. High $AFM_1$ incidence in milk and milk products can create an important public health risk due to the fact that milk and milk products are consumed widely by all age groups and especially infants, children and old aged people (Madali *et al.*, 2018). The occurrence and incidence of $AFM_1$ contamination in milk and dairy products may vary according to individual, localities and also on agricultural practices (Prandini *et al.*, 2009). Consumption of high amounts of concentrated feeds by high-yielding cows might result in high level of aflatoxin $M_1$ contamination in milk (Boukhari *et al.*, 2017). Geographical variation in the concentration of $AFM_1$ has also been reported (Bilandzic *et al.*, 2017; Ansari *et al.*, 2019).

Since $AFM_1$ has carcinogenic potency as high as that of aflatoxin $B_1$ (Henry *et al.*, 2001) thus many countries have set maximum acceptable levels for $AFM_1$ in milk and dairy products. US Food and Drug Administration (USFDA) has set a maximum permissible level of 0.5 µg/Kg of $AFM_1$ while in some European countries (EC), the maximum acceptable level is 0.05µg/kg (Van Egmond *et al.*, 1997). In order to maintain this limit, aflatoxin $B_1$ level in feeds for dairy animals must be kept limited (Patterson, 1998).

The presence of $AFM_1$ need to be considered as great human health risk and never it should be underestimated or neglected due to the unpredictability of climatic and environmental conditions and the unavailability of certain agricultural systems (characterized by poor economic conditions and/or lack of knowledge) to manage and mitigate aflatoxin contamination. According to a worldwide survey made by FAO (2015), cow milk is the main milk type used for human consumption which corresponds to 83% of world milk production, followed by buffalo milk (13%), goat milk (2%), sheep milk (1%) and camel milk (0.3%). As a result of this worldwide situation, the objective of our work was to access the levels of aflatoxin $AFM_1$ contamination in the cattle milk/ milk products of Bhagalpur, Bihar and also to evaluate the influence of factors such as type of cattle, seasons and regions/ localities on the prevalence of aflatoxin $M_1$ contamination in milk in order to develop future strategies for prevention/ control.

In case of milk samples, maximum aflatoxin $M_1$ contamination occurred in cow milk (58%) followed by buffalo milk (52%), however, the least per cent contamination was obtained in Sudha milk samples (25%). The result was in conformity with the previous work (Hussain *et al.*, 2010) in which they analyzed 55,40, 30, 24 and 20 milk samples of buffaloes, cows, goats, sheep and camel for $AFM_1$ and contamination level was 34.5%. 37.5%, 20% and 16.7%, respectively. Previous work from abroad have reported that the percentage of $AFM_1$ contamination in cow milk was more (78.8%) than other milk whereas, in water buffalo milk, camel milk, sheep milk and goat milk were 38.7%, 12.5%, 37.3% and 27.1%, respectively (Rahimi *et al.*, 2010). Several other researchers (Srivastava *et al.*, 2001; Ghanem and Orfi, 2009; Hassan and Kassaify, 2014) have also reported the presence of high per cent of $AFM_1$ contamination in cow milk than milk of other animals. The presence of low level of $AFM_1$ in water buffalo and other cattle milk were attributed to the facts that they were fed by grazing and 3-4 months stored grains (Nile *et al.*, 2015). Several scientists have reported the presence of higher concentration of *Lactobacilli* in buffalo milk (than cow milk), which bind to $AFB_1$ and $AFM_1$ which thereby, decontaminate the secreted milk (Oatley *et al.*, 2000; Pierides *et al.*, 2000; Peltonen *et al.*, 2001; Rahimi *et al.*, 2010). Cow milk has comparatively higher protein content (whey protein) than buffalo milk (Cozma *et al.*, 2011).

In our investigations, out of 182 milk samples of milk analyzed, only one sample of milk contained aflatoxin $M_1$ exceeding 0.5µg/kg. In 29 samples, the toxin range was in between 0.05 µg/kg, however, remaining samples contained amount less than 0.05 µg/kg. To achieve the objective to maintain the minimal permissible level of toxin, aflatoxin $B_1$ level in feeds for dairy animals must be limited to keep levels of $AFM_1$ in milk <0.05 µg/kg (Patterson, 1998). In previous works, aflatoxin $M_1$ contamination was observed in camel and cow milk (Gurbay *et al.*, 2006; Boudra *et al.*, 2007; Rahimi *et al.*, 2010; Elzupir *et al.*, 2010). Occurrence of aflatoxin $M_1$ in goat milk has also been reported (Virdis *et al.*, 2008). Aflatoxin $M_1$ has also been reported in sheep milk (Battacone *et al.*, 2005). Comparatively high levels (Mean value 0.027ppm) of aflatoxin $M_1$ has been reported in earlier work while working on cow milk (Ansari *et al.*, 2019). Concentration of aflatoxin $M_1$ in Sudha dairy milk, milk powder, cheese and milk shake samples were less than 0.05 µg/kg, mean of 0.013 ± 0.004, 0.013 ± 0.012, 0.013 ± 0.011 and 0.014 µg/kg, respectively. In our study, Sudha dairy milk (which was pasteurized milk) showed less risk of $AFM_1$ toxin than fresh milk of cow, buffalo and goat. Our results are in conformity with the earlier work that raw milk contained more aflatoxin level than pasteurized and UHT (Ultra high temperature processed) milk (Zheng *et al.*, 2013; Rama *et al.*, 2015). The explanation to our findings is that the pasteurized milk is being stored in refrigerator, however, the raw milk is kept at room temperature. At UHT there are the reports of detoxification of aflatoxin (Fallah, 2010). It is known that aflatoxin level does not increase at 4°C or below temperatures but its level increases in optimum room temperatures due to secondary contamination (Galvano *et al.*, 1996). $AFM_1$ in milk can be reduced by good manufacturing, transporting and storage practices. For food safety purposes, there is a need for quality control during processing and distribution of those products (Deveci, 2007; Boukhari *et al.*, 2017).

### Regional Variation of Aflatoxin $M_1$ in Milk of Different Cattle

While considering the type of cattle and the regions, it was found that maximum contamination (58%) of milk was in cow milk of urban areas, followed by buffalo (52%) and goat milk (48%). In semi-urban area the contamination of aflatoxin $M_1$ was comparatively higher than the rural areas. However, in rural areas contamination percentage was lower than semi-urban and urban areas. Maximum concentration of aflatoxin $M_1$ was obtained from buffalo milk of urban area (mean = 0.126µg/kg) followed by cow milk of urban area (0.105µg/kg). In rural and semi-urban areas cattles are fed with freshly harvested feed and/ or by grazing, where the chances of aflatoxin $B_1$ contamination level was comparatively low.

However, during the spring, summer and monsoons there was non-significant differences with respect to the levels of aflatoxins $M_1$. Mean value of aflatoxin $M_1$ in winter season was significantly low (0.030 µg/kg) compared to spring and monsoon seasons. Our results are in contrary to the previous works (Tahoun *et al.*, 2017; Mazafari *et al.*, 2017), who revealed that the levels of $AFB_1$ and $AFM_1$ in feedstuff and milk were maximum during winter followed by autumn, spring and summer. Seasonal and geographical effects are factors which have pronounced influence on the level of $AFM_1$ (Tajkarimi *et al.*, 2008; Choudhary *et al.*, 2020). High temperature and high humidity prevailing in this locality during spring, summer and monsoons provided ideal conditions for *A. flavus* infestation and aflatoxin synthesis. Once the food/ feed ingredients get infested, aflatoxin enters into the food chain (Diener *et al.*, 1987; Sinha and Choudhary, 2008; Choudhary *et al.*, 2020). Aflatoxin $M_1$ can be minimized through good preharvest (crop rotation, irrigation, fungal resistance, biological control) during harvest (ripening, dry matter) and post harvest (storage, cooling, dryness, processing etc.) management of feed crops. Aflatoxin contamination can occur in milk and milk products either through carry-over of aflatoxin $B_1$ from feed to milk by cattle or by secondary contamination with *Aspergillus flavus*. Per cent contamination of aflatoxin was comparatively high in cow raw milk of urban areas followed by buffalo milk, however, the level of contamination in most of the samples was within the regulatory limits (USFDA, EU and CAC).

## B. Carry-over of Aflatoxin from Cattle Feed ($AFB_1$) to Milk ($AFM_1$).

Large differences in mean carry-over rate of aflatoxin between cows of early (two to four week after calving) and late (34 to 36 weeks after calving) lactation periods were observed. The difference in the carry-over rate between early and late lactation was about a factor of 3.3. Our work was in conformity with the findings of previous workers (Lafont *et al.*, 1980), who observed a factor of 3.5 as a difference of carry-over in early and late lactating cows. An important part of this difference in carry-over can be explained by the milk yield as in early lactating period there was comparatively higher milk yield (20.1 kg/day). $AFM_1$ concentration in milk in early lactation period also contributed to the higher carry-over. The results of per cent aflatoxin carry-over of individual cows in early and late lactation are shown in Tables - 11 and 12 indicating differences in aflatoxin excretion in milk between cows of the same stage of lactation despite their similar aflatoxin $B_1$ intake. High milk-yielding cows had a higher carry-over rate than low milk-yielding cows, however, with the same $AFB_1$ intake. The $AFM_1$ content of milk must be related to the $AFM_1$ in blood concentration, as the supply of nutrients for milk synthesis is a carry-over process of molecules from the blood to the alveolar cells of the mammary gland (Veldman *et al.,* 1992; Britzi *et al.,* 2013). The $AFM_1$ in blood concentration in its turn is dependent on the amount of $AFB_1$ absorbed from the intestinal tract, the $AFB_1$ liver conversion to $AFM_1$ and the $AFM_1$ excretion in urine, bile and milk (Masoero *et al.,* 2007). An explanation for the difference in aflatoxin carry- over results has to include those factors. The carry-over rate of aflatoxin was independent of the $AFB_1$ intake, as determined in the intake range 34.6 to 48.9µg $AFB_1$ per cow per day. Earlier, Munksgaard *et al.* (1987) also observed high carry over rate related to high ingestion of aflatoxin $B_1$. $AFB_1$ conversion in the liver is mixed function oxidase (MFO) system which is not a rate limiting step (Steiner *et al.,* 1990; Veldman *et al.,* 1992). The discrepancy in $AFM_1$ content of milk from high and low milk-yielding cows could be due to differences in the enzyme activities of the MFO system. Besides $AFM_1$, $AFQ_1$ and $AFP_1$ are also metabolized through MFO mediated system. The direction of metabolism depends on different enzyme activities of the MFO-system. MFO-system of cows also could be induced (Hammann, 1990). Thus, conversion of $AFB_1$ to $AFM_1$ (MFO mediated system) might be the reason of variation in the $AFB_1$ carry-over. Variability in carry-over rate was also observed by Van Egmond (1989), who, however, observed that there was no relationship between milk yield and aflatoxin $M_1$ excretion. Allecroft (1968) found that cows excreted about 10 times more $AFM_1$ in urine and by way of the bile and faeces than in milk. Therefore, the amount of $AFM_1$ excreted in milk has a minor effect on the $AFM_1$ in blood concentration. In the process of milk formation about 300 to 500 litres of blood flows through the gland for the production of one litre of milk. On the other hand, it has been argued that there is a passive concentration- dependent permeability of $AFM_1$ from blood to the alveolar cells of the mammary gland resulting thereby, the relationship between carry-over and milk yield (Sumantri *et al.,* 2012; Britzi *et. al.,* 2013). A difference in the permeability of the alveolar cell membranes themselves could be a cause of variation in $AFB_1$ carry-over (Veldman *et al.,* 1992). It has been reported that bacterial (Staphylococcus) infected udder in cows secreted elevated level of $AFM_1$. Udder condition appears to be another cause of variations, as udder infections may cause increase permeability. Increased udder permeability in early lactation could also be a reason for the higher $AFM_1$ content of milk of cows at 2 to 4 weeks in lactation. In addition to the animal factors, the analytical precision of the $AFB_1$ and $AFM_1$ determinations can also be taken into account. The within-laboratory variation for the HPLC method for $AFB_1$ at a level of 10 µg/kg food and for $AFM_1$ at a level of 0.03 µg/kg milk is proportionately 0.11 and 0.08, respectively. These uncertainties in $AFB_1$ and $AFM_1$ measurements may contribute to the variations in carry- over rates. In our investigations we found that high carry-over rate of $AFM_1$

was directly correlated to the high ingestion of $AFB_1$ due to higher consumption of feed. Aflatoxin $M_1$ carry over within the cattle body is influenced by the factors like the amount of $AFB_1$ ingestion, its absorption from intestinal tract, $AFB_1$ conversion to $AFM_1$ in liver cell and its excretion in urine, bile and milk (Masoero *et al.*, 2007). Large variations between individual dairy cows were observed and with varying carry-over rate. Kiermeier *et al.* (1975) reported high difference (6.75 times) in carry-over rate among different cows. Their results showed that the carry-over rate was linearly correlated with milk yield and can be expressed by the equation: carry-over rate = amount of milk yield per cow per day + 0.013 (r = 0.80). At a milk yield of 18.2 kg/day the carry-over rate was around 0.025 (Van Egmond, 1989).

## C. Influence of Different Variables in the Carryover Rate of Aflatoxin

### C1. Influence of Seasons

Among the seasons, wet season of monsoons showed comparatively higher range of natural intake of $AFB_1$ and $AFM_1$ excretion, which in turn influenced the carry-over rate. $AFB_1$ intake during this season was 23.4µg/ day to 64.8µg/day, with an average value of 42.2 ± 0.96µg/day. An average of 2.68 ± 2.28 µg $AFM_1$ was excreted on each day during the wet seasons. The carry-over rate during monsoon was recorded 0.063 ± 0.008. The lowest carry-over rate was observed during winters. Several reports from different countries are available related to the influence of seasons on $AFB_1$ uptake and $AFM_1$ excretion in milk (Asi *et al.*, 2012; Xiong *et al.*, 2013; Bilandzin *et al.*, 2014). There was elevated concentration of $AFM_1$ in milk in dry/ winter periods, which were influenced by use of greater amounts of mixed supplementary feedstuffs and corn contaminated with high levels of $AFB_1$. Nemati *et al.* (2010) reported significantly lower levels of mean $AFM_1$ level in summer and autumn compared to winter and spring seasons. Raw milk samples during different seasons were evaluated (Xiong *et al.*, 2013) and significantly high ($p<0.05$) levels of $AFM_1$ was observed during winters compared to the rest other samples. Morning milk has been reported to contain higher percentage of toxin than evening milk. Lack of activities of cow has been attributed to be the reason for higher percentage of toxin in morning milk (Hussain and Anwar, 2008). The possible reason behind the higher $AFM_1$ in winter in those regions has been attributed to favourable temperature and moisture for toxin production in harvested and stored feed. In winters mostly milking animals are fed with compound feeds and thus enhances $AFM_1$ concentration in milk (Aplebaun *et al.*, 1982; Blanco *et al.*, 1988; Bilandzic *et al.*, 2010; Mahmoudi and Norian, 2015). Bahrami *et al.* (2016) from Iran also reported significantly higher levels ($p<0.05$) of aflatoxins in winters. They concluded that in winter season animal feeds were stored at inappropriate conditions which lead to the growth of aflatoxigenic moulds and aflatoxins.

In our locality, high temperature (25.45%) and high relative humidity (>80%) prevailed during monsoons, which lead to excessive moulding of cattle feed with aflatoxigenic strains of *A. flavus*. Any attempt to reduce $AFM_1$ in milk should focus on reduction in the level of $AFB_1$ in cattle feed as a linear relationship have been established between the concentration of $AFM_1$ in milk and $AFB_1$ consumed in feed. Moreover, $AFB_1$ contamination in feed is influenced by agro-climatic conditions of specific locality/ region as well as preharvest, during harvest and post harvest conditions of feeds.

## C2. Influence of Cow Age on Carry Over Rate of Aflatoxin

For age factors, the lactation (calving cycle) of the cows were considered. The carry-over rate of aflatoxin from $AFB_1$ to $AFM_1$ was studied during different milking stages i.e. first, third and fourth lactation periods (after $1^{st}$, $3^{rd}$ and $4^{th}$ calving of the same cows). During the first lactation, the range of milk yield was 11.7 to 14.3 kg/day (Mean = 12.9 ± 0.91 kg/day) and the average range of $AFM_1$ contamination was 0.045 ± 0.003µg/kg, with the mean carry-over rate of 0.042 ± 0.004. By the time those cows reached the third calving stage, the dietary feed intake of cows (kg/day) had increased by almost 4-5 kgs rendering thereby, the mean uptake of $AFB_1$ as 36.9 ± 0.97µg/day (compared to 35.6 ± 0.67µg/day during first calving stage). The mean value of milk yield also increased from 12.9 ± 0.91kg/ day to 16.4 ± 1.41kg/day during third stage of calving. The carry-over rate in third calving stage was recorded 0.048 ± 0.004 (slightly higher than first lactating cycle). The experimental subjects (cows) were kept same in order to maintain consistency in the physiological state (an independent variable) of metabolism.

In our investigation, it has been observed that with the increase in the intake of feed, the milk yield increased and thereby, there was resultant increase in carryover of aflatoxin. Previous workers (Lafont *et al.*, 1980; Price *et al.*, 1985 and Masoero *et al.*, 2007) have stated that high milk yield was the main factor contributing to increased carry-over of aflatoxin. Increased milk yield had direct correlation with the stages of lactation (Britzi *et al.*, 2013). Fink-Gremmels (2008) observed that at the same rate of $AFB_1$ ingestion (even after the increased uptake of dietary feed), milk yield and carry-over rate increased due to increase in liver biotransformation and digestion rate. Further, he found that the excretion of $AFM_1$ varied from one milking cycle to another milking cycle.

During fourth calving stage, the average production of milk decreased to 14.3 ± 1.27kg/day from (16.4 ± 1.41kg/day), however, dietary intake of $AFB_1$ increased during fourth lactation cycle (37.1 ± 0.67µg/day) than third lactation cycle (36.9 ± 0.97µg/day). The mean value of $AFM_1$ excretion in milk of cows during fourth lactation cycle was 0.048 ± 0.002µg/kg (1.61 ± 0.24µg/day) with the carry-over rate of 0.043 ± 0.005. The average value of $AFM_1$ excretion was maximum during third lactating cycle (0.049 ± 0.002 µg/kg) followed by fourth lactating cycle (0.048 ± 0.002µg/kg), however, it was the lowest (0.045 ± 0.003µg/kg) in first lactating cycle. Our findings supported the earlier works (Frobish, 1986; Diaz, 2004; Masoero, 2007; Battacone, 2003) related to lactation stages, milk yields and carry-over rate of cows. Their studies suggested that during the period (few hours to few days) of maximum milk yield, the carryover rate was also high. The decrease in carryover during fourth lactating stage can be correlated with the study of Miller and Wilson (1994), who opined that aflatoxin metabolism start from rumen of the cattle and being carried out by hepatic system, which gets weakened with the age. Kiessling *et al.* (1984) and Saltzmann *et al.* (2019) suggested that the types of microbiota in the rumen of the cattle also determined the level of degradation of aflatoxin, however, their incidence varied with the age. Masoero *et al.* (2007) and Allecroft (1968) found that the concentration of $AFM_1$ depended on the amount of $AFB_1$ conversion to $AFM_1$ in liver and its excretion in urine, bile and milk. In our observations we found that in fourth calving stage the amount of dietary intake of $AFB_1$ increased, however, $AFM_1$ concentration in milk decreased. The discharge of $AFM_1$ through urine and bile might have increased, thereby reducing its detection in milk (as in cows urine detects 10 times more $AFM_1$ as compared to milk) (Allecroft, 1968). Moreover, with the age of cows, their physiology and metabolic activities gets weakened. The excretion of $AFM_1$ in milk is a passive, concentration dependent permeability from blood to the alveolar cells of mammary gland, thereby directly influencing the milk yield and carry-over rate (Sumantri *et al.*, 2012; Britzi *et. al.*, 2013). Moreover, the possibilities of degradation of aflatoxin through rumen microbiota cannot be ruled out. If there is the less excretion of toxin, the possibilities of toxic effects on vital organs of cattle cannot be ruled out (Sinha and Choudhary, 2008).

### C3. Influence of Individual of Breeds on Carry-Over of Aflatoxin

Nine breeds of cows (Jersey, Sahiwal, Holstein friesein, Bachaur, Gangaitri, Gir, Harynavi, Red Sindhi and Taylor) were selected to test their capabilities for $AFM_1$ excretion level in milk. Average intake of the quantity of foods (TMR) by those breeds varied from 13 kgs – 17 kgs. Gir, Gangaitri and Bachaur were low milk yielding cows while Holstein Friesian, Taylor and Jersey were observed as high milk yielding cows.

Remarkable variations in the carry-over rate among the cows of different breeds were observed. Taylor breed recorded the maximum (0.063 ± 0.007) carry-over of aflatoxin followed by Holstein Friesian (0.051 ± 0.007). Haryanavi and Jersey showed carry-over rate of 0.041 ± 0.007 and 0.038 ± 0.004, respectively. In Red Sindhi the carry-over rate of aflatoxin was 0.039 ± 0.008 with lower milk yield (9.7 ± 0.89 kg/day) Sahiwal, Gangaitri, Baichur had comparatively the lower carry-over 0.032 ± 0.004, 0.029 ± 0.003 and 0.027 ± 0.010, respectively. Gir breed of cow recorded the lowest carry-over rate (0.023 ± 0011) and also had the lowest milk yield (4.5 ± 1.78kg/day).

From the perspective of milk yield, it was evident that Holstein Friesian, Taylor, Jersey and Haryanvi were high milk yielding cows, however, Red Sindhi, Sahiwal, Gangaitri, bachaur and Gir fell under the category of medium and low milk yielding cows. Our findings of carry-over rate are in conformity with the previous work of Lafont *et al.* (1980); Munksgaard *et al.* (1987) and Patterson *et al.*

(1989), who observed that high milk yielding cows metabolized comparatively higher amounts of $AFB_1$ to $AFM_1$ than low milk yielding cows. However, the variation among high milking or low milking cows can be supported with the fact that carry-over of aflatoxin to a large extent depends upon the dietary intake (Frobish *et al.*, 1986). High milk yielding cows had comparatively higher feed uptake and thereby, they had more ingestion of $AFB_1$ through feed. Moreover, the cows under investigation were raised by different cattle dwellers and hence, the difference in type of feed as well as the hygienic conditions adopted by the breeders varied. This fact supported the reason for the variation among Taylor and Holstein Friesian breed, wherein milk yield by Holstein Friesian was more compared to Taylor, however, carry-over rate was lower. Earlier workers (Gaili *et al.*, 2000; Khaskheli *et al.*, 2005; Dowelmadina *et al.*, 2014; Mohamed Elhassan *et al.*, 2015) reported that the variation in the toxin component in the milk of camels was dependent upon the breeds of lactating camels. Sahin *et al.* (2016) attributed the variation of $AFM_1$ level of milk samples to the genetic variation among dairy cows apart from other factors such as geographical and seasonal variations.

Britzi *et al.* (2013) observed that one of the eight cows had exceptionally high carry-over rate (155.3%), which was above the mean. They suggested that it may occur naturally in dairy cow genetic pool, where individual with high carry-over rate can develop. The feed ingested by different breeds of cows were in the range of 13 - 22 kgs/ day. The breed of cows with higher milk yield had more food being metabolized into milk, thereby there were the chances of more $AFB_1$ (along with feed). The conversion of $AFB_1$ into $AFM_1$ takes place in the liver of cows and it is a vital process which varies with the individuals. Another possible reason may be that the breeds with low milk yield might have more $AFB_1$ passing through urine, bile or dung (faeces) or with less capability of $AFB_1$ conversion to milk toxin. Volkel *et al.* (2011) suggested that the amount of $AFM_1$ excreted was dependent upon the $AFB_1$ intake (with the feed) per kg body weight. The variation of carry-over within the species and breeds earlier has also been reported by different researchers (Walte *et al.*, 2016). Makun *et al.* (2017) in their experiments found wherein the aflatoxin $M_1$ in the liver samples of cows in the range of 0.000 – 21.730µg/kg, which, however, had the great variation among the individuals.

## D. Aflatoxin Level in Milk Components

The lactose and protein (of SNF), fat, water and minerals in full cream were present at an average value of 4.36 ± 0.02 and 4.64 ± 0.07, 6.01 ± 0.03 and 84.91 ± 0.02 per cent, respectively of total milk constituents. The SNFs in toned, double toned and skimmed milk were nearly similar, however, the quantity of fat was remarkably different.

Variations in fat per cent of the raw milk, full cream, toned, double-toned and skimmed milk and the corresponding variations in $AFM_1$ concentrations (in different processed/ unprocessed milk) were observed. The content of fat in raw milk was 3.61 % and the mean value of $AFM_1$ concentration was

0.043 ± 0.005µg/kg. However, toned milk, double-toned and skimmed milk showed reduction in the mean value of $AFM_1$ concentration as 0.041 ± 0.006, 0.038 ± 0.001, 0.014 ± 0.011µg/kg, respectively, with the corresponding decrease in fat concentration in those milk types. Full-cream milk showed the highest fat per cent (6.01 ± 0.03) compared to other types of milk and also maximum $AFM_1$ concentration value 0.044 ± 0.002µg/kg, which, however, was within the EU limit. This variation can be understood with the fact that extra fat added to the raw milk was saturated processed fat, which was mixed in fixed proportion in order to maintain the desired quality of milk. Our findings supported the previous reports (Yiannikouris and Jouany, 2002; Kalac, 2011; Becker-Algeri *et al.*, 2016) who suggested that the level of aflatoxin excretion in milk was affected by its lipophilicity characteristics. Earlier Langat *et al.* (2016) also observed that the processed milk showed comparatively low level of aflatoxin contamination compared to raw milk.

However, unlike the components of milk, the fat constituents of dairy products showed no relation with the $AFM_1$ concentration in milk. The fat concentration in butter was maximum (80%) among all the dairy products studied, however, the $AFM_1$ concentration was 0.213 ± 0.05µg/kg. Likewise, fat concentration of khoya was 36.9 per cent and $AFM_1$ concentration varied from 0.234µg/kg to 0.624 µg/kg. Previously, Seagun *et al.* (2008) observed higher $AFM_1$ concentration in cheeses compared to milk. Ardic *et al.* (2009) observed the $AFM_1$ concentration in cheese to be 5 fold as comparison to the milk from which it was produced. The increase in $AFM_1$ concentration had been attributed to the concentrated product of milk. Further, it was observed that the fat content of dairy products had no correlation with the $AFM_1$ variations. It was also observed by Seagun *et al.* (2008) who inferred that the affinity of $AFM_1$ for the casein leads to the increase in aflatoxin $M_1$ concentration. The products like khoya, paneer, cheese have comparatively higher content of protein compared to raw milk. The findings of Ikins (1986) stated close association between milk protein and $AFM_1$. The report further stated that cheese was mainly protein and if prepared from contaminated milk would contain higher concentration of $AFM_1$ than original milk. Govaris *et al.* (2002) reported that high per cent of *Lactobacillus* decreased $AFM_1$ concentration in milk. This might be the reason that we observed lower level of $AFM_1$ in curd. Prandini *et al.* (2007) suggested that $AFM_1$ remained soluble in aqueous phase of milk suggesting thereby, that after removal of water the $AFM_1$ content was more in concentrated matter.

## E. Approaches to Control Aflatoxin in Cattle Feed

The primary approaches for control of aflatoxin contamination can be made through preventive measures. Following the HACCP approaches various check points to control the infection of *A. flavus* and aflatoxin synthesis during preharvest, harvest, transport, storage and processing systems can be made. There are several reports with regard to the control of aflatoxins through HACCP practices (Choudhary and Sinha, 2008; Toregeani-Mendes *at al.*, 2011)

## Use of Plant Extracts, Commercial Phenol, Volatile Organic Compounds

Through the application of plant extracts, phenolics and volatile organic compounds, there was 20-83% inhibition of $AFB_1$ contents in mixed total ration (MTR) of cattle. The organic volatile compound (acetic acid) showed the maximum reduction (83.1%) in aflatoxin contamination. Among the wild plant extracts, *Azadirachta indica* A. Juss. showed the maximum per cent reduction (52.4%) in $AFB_1$, followed by volatile compound, Propionic acid (39.1%). Formaldehyde resulted in 38.2% inhibition of aflatoxin synthesis in the composite cattle feed substrates. In case of treatment with the herbal extracts of *Thuja orientalis* L., *Ocimum sanctum* L. and *Ricinus communis* L., the inhibition per cent were 29.5, 25.1 and 23.7, respectively. Commercial phenolics (Tannic acid) showed the least reduction (20.4%) in aflatoxin synthesis. The plant extracts are known for antifungal activities and thereby, reducing aflatoxins synthesis as they have ability to inhibit infection inducing molecules (Kazemi *et al.*, 2017). Our result of aflatoxin reduction by acetic acid supported the previous work of Reddy *et al.* (1983) who observed 83.3 per cent reduction in growth of *A. flavus* and complete suppression of the aflatoxin production. The inhibitory effect of neem extract on aflatoxin synthesis was in coherence with the work of Bhatnagar *et al.* (1988) wherein, they observed that 10% neem extract (v/v) checked the fungal growth by 98% and also inhibited the aflatoxin production. With the increase in the concentration of neem extract (20%) they further observed an irreversible inhibition of *A. parasiticus*. Even if mycelia were removed from neem extract, the aflatoxin synthesis was not restored. Previous work of Bhatnagar *et al.* (1987) showed that the early precursors (Averantin and Norsolorinic acid) of aflatoxin $B_1$ were not formed in neem extract treated mycelia, although the enzymes for their synthesis were present. Precursors Averantin and Sterigmatocystin get converted to $AFB_2$ (less toxic aflatoxin). Further, formaldehyde and propionic acid showed the mycelia inhibition and aflatoxin production in medium range. The inhibitory effect of aldehydes and other volatile organic compounds was due to interaction of those substances with the enzyme system of the fungus (Nyman, 1969). Similarly, Beckwith *et al.* (1976) had also observed the chemical inactivation of aflatoxins while using acids and bases.

Earlier Singh *et al.* (1983) had also observed 47% reduction of aflatoxin in maize, 66.67 on groundnut and 50% on rice while treating with the *Euphorbia hirta* L., using maize as substrate.

The effects of different types of lights were also observed on the production of $AFB_1$ on maize grains (a major ingredient of cattle feed). Tubelight showed the minimum (2%) reduction of aflatoxins followed by bulb light (4%). UV light showed the maximum reduction (23%) of aflatoxin $B_1$ in maize grains. Sun dried maize grains showed 12% reduction in aflatoxin $B_1$ contents. Earlier, Shantha and Sreenivasamurthy (1977) recorded 99% reduction of aflatoxin through sun-light treatment, using groundnut oil as substrate. In earlier work from our laboratory, Bilgrami *et al.* (1984) suggested the sunlight treatment for mass scale detoxification of aflatoxins in feed substrates.

## Use of Activated Carbon to Reduce the Aflatoxin Carry-over in Milk

Five test cows in the first week were fed with normal feed which, however, contained aflatoxin $B_1$ (control set of experiment). The $AFM_1$ excretion and carry-over rate were observed of those cows. Activated carbon was used as supplement with dietary intake of cows, as it had been earlier proved as nontoxic absorbent of aflatoxin (Cooney, 1980). With the intake of activated carbon (2%), the remarkable reduction in carryover rate of aflatoxin has earlier also been reported (Harvey *et al.*, 1991; Galvano *et al.*, 1996; Soha *et al.*, 2007). Galvano *et al.* (1996) found high affinity of activated carbon to $AFB_1$. Reduction in carry-over rate was observed in the range of 15.9 to 44.4 per cent. Our investigation was in accordance with the result obtained by Smith *et al.* (1994) wherein, they observed reduction of approximately 36% aflatoxin content when feed was supplemented with activated carbon.

## Processing of Milk

Ultra-heating (UHT) performed at 140 C for 3 seconds showed the maximum reduction (41.46%) in the $AFM_1$ content of milk. The $AFM_1$ content in raw milk samples (which were subjected to different heating conditions) was 0.041µg/kg and post UHT, the level of aflatoxin $M_1$ content was 0.024 ± 0.009µg/kg. Previous studies (Zheng *et al.*, 2013 and Rama *et al.*, 2015) revealed that $AFM_1$ level was the lowest when treated with UHT milk. The sudden high temperature kills various bacteria and fungus including spores. The processed milks are stored in refrigerator temperature which eventually restricts the growth of aflatoxin (Kanungo *et al.*, 2014). After UHT, temperature treatment at 121°C for 20 mins the level of $AFM_1$ content was 0.026 ± 0.006µg/kg. According to the study carried out by Choudhary *et al.* (1998), sterilization at 121°C for 15 mins showed degradation in $AFM_1$ content by 12.21%. The temperature rise between 75°C to 100°C showed no notable reduction, however, continuous heating at fixed temperature of 100°C for 30 mins led the reduction from 0.033 ± 0.007µg/kg to 0.031 ± 0.002µg/kg. It was also conferred that the destruction of $AFM_1$ depended on the temperature and time combination of the treatment given (Choudhary *et al.*, 1998). Sinha (1998) showed reduction in $AFM_1$ contamination by 7.62% after pasteurization of milk, the result was in conformity of my findings. Govaris *et al.* (2001) also reported that partial degradation of $AFM_1$ through pasteurization temperature.

CHAPTER 5

# Summary

The incidence and diversity of moulds in the cattle feed were recorded in the agro-climatic conditions and varied seasons of Bhagalpur. Maximum incidence (87%) of *A. flavus* was observed in the monsoons followed by summer (76%). Winters, however, showed the least occurrence of *A. flavus* (19%).

Amount of toxins in household stored feed was found significantly high ($p<0.05\%$) compared to commercial or fresh feed samples. 33% of household stored feeds contained aflatoxin $B_1$ level higher than the upper limit of European Union (EU). In a combined observation considering different samples and various seasons in concert, the maximum aflatoxin $B_1$ level was observed in household stored cattle feeds during wet seasons, followed by commercially available feeds. During winters, comparatively lower level of aflatoxin $B_1$ was observed in freshly harvested cattle feed. It was inferred that the freshly harvested cattle feeds were relatively secured for cattle consumption as 83-95% of the samples were observed containing aflatoxin level below the EU limit (0.05μg/kg).

Poor and unhealthy management of drying of feeds were observed especially in household storage of cattle feeds. Unseasonal rain was the recurrent feature of this terrain, which resulted high moistening of the feed and thereby, providing congenial conditions for *A. flavus* infestation and aflatoxin synthesis. Freshly harvested feeds contained least content of aflatoxin while considering the three sources of feeds. Chances of aflatoxin poisoning in cattle can be minimized through feeding the cattle with fresh fodder.

Among different seasons, monsoons had shown significantly high level of ($p<0.05$) of aflatoxin contamination in the three localities under observations for all the different types of feeds of cattle. Per cent viable conidia of toxigenic *A. flavus* in wet months (monsoons) were comparatively higher than in winters or summers. In this area the high temperature, % RH and outdated storage system prevailed, which provided an ideal condition for *A. flavus* infection and aflatoxin production.

With consideration of the localities, cattle feed obtained from Naugachia had the maximum mean level of aflatoxin in every season. The mean value of aflatoxin level in cattle feed of Naugachia was 4.2 ± 1.56μg/kg followed by Bhagalpur (3.7 ± 1.45μg/kg) and Banka (3.5 ± 1.43). In this areas, flood is the recurrent feature where maize (a major ingredients of cattle feed) is harvested mostly during late August/ early September by that time crops get submerged with flood water. Farmers have no option but to harvest the crops before full maturity and thereby, kernels contained high moisture contents. Further processing (peeling, shelling and drying) of the crops are made on nearby National Highway. Frequent rains result in late drying of kernels. Such situations provided an ideal situation for *A. flavus* contamination and aflatoxin synthesis. Those contaminated maize kernels when mixed with the cattle feed, resulted in contamination of entire feed lots.

Among the raw milk samples, maximum contamination (58%) occurred in cow milk followed by buffalo (52%) however, minimum contamination (25%) of aflatoxin $M_1$ was observed in Sudha milk. 53.8% in per cent local made milk product khoya was contaminated with aflatoxin $M_1$ which was followed by curd (45%). Cheese and milkshakes were less contaminated by aflatoxin $M_1$, 25% and 28.5%, respectively. The quantitative analysis of aflatoxin $M_1$ revealed that range of aflatoxin was high in buffalo milk followed by cow milk samples. Concentration of aflatoxin $M_1$ in Sudha dairy milk, milk powder, cheese and milk shake samples were less than 0.05 μg/kg. In our study, Sudha dairy milk (which was pasteurized milk) showed less risk of $AFM_1$ than fresh milk of cow, buffalo and goat.

Considering all types of cattle, maximum contamination (58%) of aflatoxin $M_1$ occurred in milk of urban areas cow milk followed by buffalo (52%) and goat milk (48%). However, in the milk samples of rural areas per cent contamination was comparatively less than semi urban and urban area where 36% samples in milk from buffaloes were positive to aflatoxin $AFM_1$ followed by 32% from cow and goat. In rural areas farmers/ cattle breeders use to leave their cattle for grazing of fresh green grasses. They also fed their cattle with fresh fodder, whose availability was mainly season dependent.

The observation revealed that the aflatoxin $M_1$ contamination was significantly high in monsoons and spring seasons compared to winter season. Among different seasons, winter milk samples of different cattle milk showed less contamination than spring, summer and monsoons. Seasonal and geographical effects are factors which have pronounced influence in the level of $AFM_1$. High temperature and high humidity prevailing in this locality during spring, summer and monsoons provided ideal conditions for *A. flavus* infestation and aflatoxin synthesis. Once the food/ feed ingredients get infested, aflatoxin enters into the food chain.

Remarkable differences were found in the carry over rate of aflatoxin between early lactation to that of late lactation period of milking. While comparing two different lactating periods, the difference of carryover rate was found in a factor of 3.2. Variations in $AFM_1$ excretion were observed among the cows of same stage, consuming approximately similar concentrations of $AFB_1$. Rate of carry-over of $AFM_1$, however, varied among high yielding and low yielding cows. The carry-over rate varied by the factor of 1.02 among the high milk yielding cows. In case of low milk yielding cows, the carry-over rate varied by the factor of 1.04. Since the carry over factors were nearly similar and thereby, they supported a linear correlation between the carry-over rate of aflatoxin with milk yield in the same cow. The linear correlation has been expressed with the equation: carry-over rate = amount of milk yield per cow per day + 0.013 ($r = 0.80$). However, at milk yield of 35.8 and 43.5 kg/day, the carry-over rate was 0.058 and 0.061, respectively which exceeded the regulation limit of EU. EU regulation is based on ALARA (as low as reasonably acceptable level) principle. However, at level 10 times higher than this level (EU limit) is not considered to be harmful for human health (WHO, 2002). High milk-yielding cows had a higher carry-over rate than low milk-yielding cows, with the same $AFB_1$ intake. The $AFM_1$ content of milk might be related to the $AFM_1$ in blood concentration, as the supply of nutrients for milk synthesis is a carry-over process of molecules from the blood to the alveolar cells of the mammary gland. The $AFM_1$ in blood concentration in its turn is dependent on the amount of $AFB_1$ absorbed from the intestinal tract, the $AFB_1$ liver conversion to $AFM_1$ and the $AFM_1$ excretion in urine, bile and milk. $AFM_1$ concentration was maximum in the milk of urban areas. The carry-over rate of aflatoxin contamination from $AFB_1$ to $AFM_1$ was also found slightly higher in urban areas which was followed by semi-urban.

Carry-over rate of aflatoxin in milk was found to be influenced with the seasons. Wet period of monsoons showed comparatively higher range in natural intake of $AFB_1$ and $AFM_1$ excretion which also influenced the carry-over rate. From the mean data calculated for carry-over rate of all seasons with respect to individual season, it was evident that the value was maximum in monsoons (0.073), which, however, was highly significant (at $p<0.05$) compared to winters (0.040). The mean value of carry-over recorded during summer (0.054) was also significantly high to the mean value of carry-over rate of winter. However, the mean carryover rate during summer was at par with that of monsoons. The maximum carry-over rate was observed during the months of monsoons (July, August, September) where the peak values were 0.058, 0.060 and 0.073, respectively. Levels of contaimination in some of the samples, exceeded the EU limit. However, for rest of the months of year, the $AFM_1$ concentration in milk was found within the limit. The above results indicated that the $AFM_1$ contamination in raw milk was season dependent owing to the variation in the quality and type of feed given to the cows by the cattle breeders of the local areas. In our locality, high temperature (25.45%) and high relative humidity (>80%) prevailed during monsoons, which lead to excessive moulding of cattle feed with aflatoxigenic strains of *A. flavus*. Any attempt to reduce $AFM_1$ in milk should focus on reduction in the level of $AFB_1$ in cattle feed as a linear relationship have been established between the concentration of $AFM_1$ in milk and $AFB_1$ consumed in feed. Moreover, $AFB_1$ contamination in feed is influenced by agroclimatic conditions of specific locality/ region as well as preharvest, during harvest and post harvest conditions of feeds.

In order to access the influence of age on carry-over rate, different lactation stages (first, third and fourth lactation stages i.e. $1^{st}$, $3^{rd}$ and $4^{th}$ calving) of the same cows were monitored. While comparing the two lactation cycles, it was observed that mean $AFB_1$ intake among cows increased because of the higher dietary intake in third lactating cycle. Compared to the first lactation cycle, there was corresponding increase in the mean value of $AFM_1$ concentration in milk among the cows of third lactation cycle. Average ingestion of $AFB_1$ by the cows during fourth lactation (calving cycle) and it's effect on the $AFM_1$ concentration/excretion and carry-over rate of toxin were also monitored. The average value of $AFM_1$ excretion was maximum during third lactating cycle (0.049 ± 0.002 µg/kg) followed by fourth lactating cycle (0.048 ± 0.002µg/kg), however, it was least in first lactating cycle (0.045 ± 0.003µg/kg). It was observed that with the increase in the intake of feed, the milk yield increased and thereby, there was resultant increase in carryover of aflatoxin. The excretion of $AFM_1$ also varied from one milking cycle to another milking cycle. The concentration of $AFM_1$ depended on the amount of $AFB_1$ conversion to $AFM_1$ in liver and its excretion in urine, bile and milk. We found that in fourth calving stage the amount of dietary intake of $AFB_1$ increased, however, $AFM_1$ concentration in milk decreased (with the increase in the age of cows). The discharge of $AFM_1$ through urine and bile might have increased, thereby reducing its detection in milk (as in cows 10 times more $AFM_1$ is detected in urine as compared to milk). Moreover, with the age of cows, their physiology and metabolic activities gets weakened. The excretion of $AFM_1$ in milk is a passive, concentration dependent permeability from blood to the alveolar cells of mammary gland, thereby directly influencing the milk yield and carry-over rate.

The carry-over rate of milk toxin showed a considerable variations among the different breeds of cows. The maximum (0.063 ± 0.005) carry-over rate was observed in the milk of Taylor breeds followed by Holstein Friesian (0.051 ± 0.007). Haryanavi and Jersey recorded the carry-over rate of 0.041 ± 0.007 and 0.038 ± 0.004, respectively which was lower as compared to the Taylor and Holstein Friesian. It was observed that the carry-over rate was related to the milk yielding capabilities of respective cows. The carry-over rate in high milk yielding cows (Holstein Friesian, Taylor and Jersey) was comparatively higher than low yielding cows (Gir, Bachaur, Gangaitri).

High milk yielding cows metabolized comparatively higher amounts of $AFB_1$ to $AFM_1$ than low milk yielding cows. However, the variation among high milking or low milking cows can be supported with the fact that carry-over of aflatoxin to a large extent depended upon the dietary intake. High milk yielding cows had comparatively higher feed uptake and thereby, they had more ingestion of $AFB_1$ through feed. Moreover, the cows under investigation were raised by different cattle dwellers and hence, the difference in type of feed as well as the hygienic conditions adopted by the breeders were marked. This fact supported the reason for the variation among Taylor and Holstein Friesian breed, wherein milk yield by Holstein Friesian was more compared to Taylor, however, carry-over rate was lower.

Variations in fat per cent of the raw milk, full cream, toned, double-toned and skimmed milk and the corresponding variations in $AFM_1$ concentrations (in different processed/ unprocessed milk) were observed. At 3.61 % of fat in raw milk, mean value of $AFM_1$ present was 0.043 ± 0.005µg/kg. However, toned milk, double-toned and skimmed milk showed reduction in the mean value of $AFM_1$ 0.041 ± 0.006, 0.038 ± 0.001, 0.014 ± 0.011µg/kg, respectively, with their corresponding decrease in fat concentration in those milk. Full-cream milk showed high fat per cent (6.01 ± 0.03) compared to other types of milk, and also there was high $AFM_1$ (0.044 ± 0.002µg/kg). This variation might be due to the fact that extra fat added to the full cream milk (saturated processed fat) was mixed in fixed proportion in order to maintain the quality of milk were responsible for high level of aflatoxin.

Unlike the types of milk, the fat constituents of dairy products showed no relation with the $AFM_1$ concentration in milk. The fat concentration of butter was maximum (80%) among all the dairy products studied, and also the $AFM_1$ concentration was high. The increase in $AFM_1$ concentration had been attributed to the concentrated product of milk. The affinity of $AFM_1$ for the casein leads to the increase in aflatoxin $M_1$ concentration. The products like khoya, paneer, cheese have comparatively higher content of protein compared to raw curd. High per cent of *Lactobacillus* decreased $AFM_1$ concentration in milk. This might be the reason that we observed lower level of $AFM_1$ in curd.

For possible control strategies, one of the possible approaches can be made by applying effective integrated aflatoxin management systems at different stages of crop management (Preharvest, harvest, transport, storage and processing systems) based on HACCP approaches. Practices such as dietary intake of fresh feeds like green grasses etc. can be given to the cows. It was observed that by feeding freshly harvested feeds/ green feeds to cows, there was comparatively least excretion of $AFM_1$ in milk.

The inhibition per cent through different treatments (with plant extracts, phenolics and volatile organic compounds) was observed in the range of 22-83% of the $AFB_1$ contents in mixed total ration (MTR) of cattle. The organic volatile compound (acetic acid) showed the maximum reduction (83.1%) in aflatoxin contamination. Among the plant extracts, *Azadirachta indiaca* A. Juss showed the maximum per cent reduction (52.4) in $AFB_1$, followed by Propionic acid. Formaldehyde resulted in 38.2% inhibition of aflatoxin synthesis in the composite cattle feed substrates. In case of treatment with the herbal extracts of *Euphorbia hirta* L., *Thuja orientalis* L., *Ocimum sanctum* L. and *Ricinus communis* L., the inhibition per cent observed were 36.8, 29.5, 25.1 and 23.7, respectively. Commercial phenolics (Tannic acid) showed the least reduction in aflatoxin contents. The early precursors (Averantin and Norsolorinic acid) of aflatoxin $B_1$ were not formed in neem extract treated mycelia. Precursors Averantin and Sterigmatocystin get converted to $AFB_2$ (less toxic aflatoxin). The inhibitory effect of aldehydes and other volatile organic compounds was due to interaction of those substances with the enzyme system of the fungus.

The effects of different lights were also observed on $AFB_1$ synthesis on maize grains. Tubelight showed the minimum reduction. UV light showed the maximum reduction (23%) of aflatoxin $B_1$ in maize. Sun dried maize grains showed 12% reduction in aflatoxin $B_1$ contents. The remarkable reduction in carryover rate of aflatoxin with the intake of activated carbon (2%) along with cattle meal was observed. The activated carbon was fed to the same cows in second week. Reduction in carry over rate was observed in the range of 15.9 to 44.4 per cent. Activated carbon was used as supplement with dietary intake of cows, as it had been earlier proved as nontoxic absorbent of aflatoxin.

Ultra-heating (UHT) performed at 140°C for 3 seconds showed the maximum reduction (41.46%) in the $AFM_1$ content of milk. The sudden high temperature is known to kill various spores of bacteria and fungus as well. After UHT, temperature treatment at 121°C for 20 minutes, the level of $AFM_1$ content was 0.026 ±0.006µg/kg. The temperature rise between 75°C to 100°C showed no reduction, however, maintaining the temperature of 100°C for 30 minutes led to the reduction from 0.033 ± 0.007µg/kg to 0.031 ± 0.002µg/kg. It was also conferred that the destruction of $AFM_1$ depended on the temperature and time combination treatments. Partial degradation of $AFM_1$ occurs through pasteurization temperature.

# Reference


1. Adekunle, A. A., & Bassir, O. (1973). The effects of aflatoxin $B_1$ and palmotoxins $B_0$ and $G_0$ on the germination and leaf colour of the cowpea (Vigna sinensis). *Mycopathologia et mycologia applicata, 51*(4), 299-305. DOI: https://doi.org/10.1007/BF02057800
2. Aldred, D., Magan, N., & Olsen, M. (2004). The use of HACCP in the control of mycotoxins: the case of cereals. *Mycotoxins in food: detection and control. Boca Raton, Fla.: CRC Press. p*, 139-73.
3. Allcroft, R., Lewis, G., Nabney, J. & Best, P. E. (1966). Metabolism of aflatoxm in sheep: excretion of the milk toxin. *Nature, Lond. 209*, 154. https://www.cabdirect.org/cabdirect/abstract/19661405479
4. Ansari, F., Pourjafar, H., & Christensen, L. (2019). A study on the aflatoxin $M_1$ rate and seasonal variation in pasteurized cow milk from northwestern Iran. *Environmental monitoring and assessment, 191*(1), 6. DOI: https://doi.org/10.1007/s10661-018-7141-1
5. Applebaum, R. S., & Marth, E. H. (1982). Fate of aflatoxin $M_1$ in cottage cheese. *Journal of Food Protection, 45*(10), 903-904. DOI: https://doi.org/10.4315/0362-028X-45.10.903
6. Ardic, M., Karakaya, Y., Atasever, M., & Adiguzel, G. (2009). Aflatoxin $M_1$ levels of Turkish white brined cheese. *Food Control, 20*(3), 196-199. DOI: https://doi.org/10.1016/j.foodcont.2008.04.003
7. Awad, E. I., Amer, I. H., Mansour, M. H., & Ismail, S. E. Y. (2014). Qualitative and quantitative detection of aflatoxin $M_1$ residues in white soft cheese. *Alexandria Journal of Veterinary Sciences, 40*(1), 119-123. DOI: 10.5455/ajvs.149489
8. Ayar, A., Sert, D., & Con, A. H. (2007). A study on the occurrence of aflatoxin in raw milk due to feeds. *Journal of Food Safety, 27*(2), 199-207. DOI: https://doi.org/10.1111/j.1745-4565.2007.00072.x
9. Bagheri, M., Ghanbarpour, R., & Alizade, H. (2014). Shiga toxin and beta-lactamases genes in *Escherichia coli* phylotypes isolated from carcasses of broiler chickens slaughtered in Iran. *International Journal of Food Microbiology, 177*, 16-20. DOI: https://doi.org/10.1016/j.ijfoodmicro.2014.02.003

10. Bahrami, R., Shahbazi, Y., & Nikousefat, Z. (2016). Aflatoxin $M_1$ in milk and traditional dairy products from west part of Iran: occurrence and seasonal variation with an emphasis on risk assessment of human exposure. *Food Control, 62*, 250-256. DOI: https://doi.org/10.1016/j.foodcont.2015.10.039

11. Bakirci, I. (2001). A study on the occurrence of aflatoxin $M_1$ in milk and milk products produced in Van province of Turkey. *Food control, 12*(1), 47-51. DOI: https://doi.org/10.1016/S0956-7135(00)00020-7

12. Barnes, J. M. (1967). Toxic fungi with special reference to aflatoxin. *Tropical Science, 9*(2), 64-74. https://www.cabdirect.org/cabdirect/abstract/19691301605

13. Battacone, G., Nudda, A., Cannas, A., Borlino, A. C., Bomboi, G., & Pulina, G. (2003). Excretion of aflatoxin $M_1$ in milk of dairy ewes treated with different doses of aflatoxin $B_1$. *Journal of Dairy Science, 86*(8), 2667-2675. DOI: https://doi.org/10.3168/jds.S0022-0302(03)73862-4

14. Battacone, G., Nudda, A., Palomba, M., Pascale, M., Nicolussi, P., & Pulina, G. (2005). Transfer of aflatoxin $B_1$ from feed to milk and from milk to curd and whey in dairy sheep fed artificially contaminated concentrates. *Journal of Dairy Science, 88*(9), 3063-3069. DOI: https://doi.org/10.3168/jds.S0022-0302(05)72987-8

15. Becha, B. B., & Devi, S. S. (2013). Aflatoxin levels in feeds and feed ingredients of livestock and poultry in Kerala. *Journal of Veterinary medicine and Animal Science, 44*, 76-78. https://journals.cvaslibrary.com/1_44_19.pdf

16. Beckwith, A. C., Vesonder, R. F., & Ciegler, A. (1976). Chemical methods investigated for detoxifying aflatoxins in foods and feeds. DOI: https://pubs.acs.org/doi/abs/10.1021/ba-1976-0149.ch004

17. Berg, T. (2003). How to establish international limits for mycotoxins in food and feed?. *Food Control, 14*(4), 219-224. DOI: https://doi.org/10.1016/S09567135(02)00021-X

18. Betina, V. (1989). *Mycotoxins. Chemical, biological and environmental aspects*. Elsevier. 438pp. https://www.cabdirect.org/cabdirect/abstract/19911208974

19. Bhat, R., Krishnamachari, K. A. V. R., Nagarajan, V., & Tilak, T. B. G. (1975). Hepatitis due to aflatoxicosis: an outbreak in western India. *The Lancet, 305*(7915), 1061-1063. DOI: https://doi.org/10.1016/S0140-6736(75)91829-2

20. Bhatnagar, D., Ehrlich, K. C., Montalbano, B. G., & Cleveland, T. E. (1998). Alteration of Different Domains in AFLR Affects Aflatoxin Pathway Metabolism in *Aspergillus parasiticus* Transformants. *Fungal Genetics and Biology, 23*(3), 279-287. DOI: https://doi.org/10.1006/fgbi.1998.1045

21. Bhatnagar, D., Linz, J. E., & Cary, J. W., (2000). Aflatoxins: biological significance and regulation of biosynthesis. *Microbial Foodborne Diseases: mechanisms of pathogenesis and toxin synthesis*, 317-361.

22. Bhatnagar, D., McCormick, S. P., Lee, L. S., & Hill, R. A. (1987). Identification of O-methylsterigmatocystin as an aflatoxin $B_1$ and $G_1$ precursor in *Aspergillus parasiticus. Applied and Environmental Microbiology*, *53*(5), 1028-1033. https://aem.asm.org/content/aem/53/5/1028.full.pdf

23. Bianchini, A., & Bullerman, L. B. (2014). MYCOTOXINS | classification. https://onlinelibrary.wiley.com/doi/abs/10.1002/9781118832790#page=104

24. Bila, V. I. (1953). Toxic fungi in the grain of grain grasses. https://agris.fao.org/agris-search/search.do?recordID=US201300210374

25. Bilandti , N., Varenina, I., & Solomun, B. (2010). Aflatoxin M1 in raw milk in Croatia. Food Control, *21*(9), 1279-1281. DOI: https://doi.org/10.1016/j.foodcont.2010.03.003

26. Biland i , N., Bo i , ., oki , M., Sedak, M., Kolanovi , B. S., Varenina, I., & Cvetni , . (2014). Assessment of aflatoxin M1 contamination in the milk of four dairy species in Croatia. *Food control*, *43*, 18-21. DOI: https://doi.org/10.1016/j.foodcont.2014.02.044

27. Biland i , N., Varenina, I., Solomun Kolanovi , B., Bo i Luburi , ., Varga, I., elje i , B., & Cvetni , . (2017). Occurrence of aflatoxin M1 in raw cow, goat and sheep milk during spring and autumn in Croatia during 2016. *Toxin Reviews*, *36*(4), 290-296. DOI: https://doi.org/10.1080/15569543.2017.1306785

28. Bilgrami K.S. & Choudhary A.K. (1997) Mycotoxin as pre – harvest contamination of agricultural crops. Deepak Bhatnagar and K.K. Sinha Eds. *Marcel dekker pub.*, New York.

29. Bilgrami K.S. and Choudhary A.K. (1998). Mycotoxins in preharvest contamination of agricultural crops. In Mycotoxins in agriculture and food safety (pp. 19-62). CRC Press.

30. Bilgrami, K. S., Ranjan, K. S., & Choudhary, A. K. (1991). Aflatoxin contamination in monocropping and mixed cropping mustard crops of Bihar. *Indian Phytopathology*, *44*(4), 529-531.

31. Bilgrami, K. S., Sahay, S. S., & Rahman, M. F. (1990). *In vivo* production of fusarial mycotoxins on wheat and maize grains. *National Academy Science Letters*, *13*(11), 405-407.

32. Blount, W. P. (1961). Turkey —X|| disease. *Turkeys*, *9*(2), 52-55. http://toxicology.usu.edu/endnote/Blount-original-Tukey-X-paper-1961.pdf

33. Bottalico, A. (1998). Fusarium diseases of cereals: species complex and related mycotoxin profiles, in Europe. *Journal of plant Pathology*, 85-103. DOI: https://www.jstor.org/stable/41997909

34. Boudra, H., Barnouin, J., Dragacci, S., & Morgavi, D. P. (2007). Aflatoxin M1 and ochratoxin A in raw bulk milk from French dairy herds. *Journal of dairy science, 90*(7), 3197-3201. DOI: https://doi.org/10.3168/jds.2006-565

35. Bokhari, F., Aly . M., Alkelany, A., & Rabah, S. (2017), Presence of aflatoxin $M_1$ in milk samples collected from Jeddah, Saudi Arabia. IOSR Jornal of Pharmacy 7(05), 99-52.

36. Brian, P. W., Dawkins, A. W., Grove, J. F., Hemming, H. G., Lowe, D., & Norris, G. L. F. (1961). Phytotoxic compounds produced by *Fusarium equiseti. Journal of experimental botany, 12*(1), 1-12. DOI: https://doi.org/10.1093/jxb/12.1.1

37. Britzi, M., Friedman, S., Miron, J., Solomon, R., Cuneah, O., Shimshoni, J. A., ... & Shlosberg, A. (2013). Carry-over of aflatoxin $B_1$ to aflatoxin $M_1$ in high yielding Israeli cows in mid-and late-lactation. *Toxins, 5*(1), 173-183. DOI: https://doi.org/10.3390/toxins5010173

38. Bryden, W. L. (2012). Food and feed, mycotoxins and the perpetual pentagram in a changing animal production environment. *Animal production science, 52*(7), 383-397. DOI: https://doi.org/10.1071/AN12073

39. Bryden, W. L. (2012). Mycotoxin contamination of the feed supply chain: Implications for animal productivity and feed security. *Animal Feed Science and Technology, 173*(1-2), 134-158. DOI: https://doi.org/10.1016/j.anifeedsci.2011.12.014

40. Cahill, S. G., Fisher, R. W., & Llewellyn, G. C. (1978). Examination and evaluation of germination and protonemal development for *Onclea sensibilis* fern spores treated with aflatoxin $B_1$. *Mycopathologia, 64*(1), 43-47. DOI: https://doi.org/10.1007/BF00443088

41. Carvajal, M., Rojo, F., Méndez, I., & Bolanos, A. (2003). Aflatoxin $B_1$ and its interconverting metabolite aflatoxicol in milk: the situation in Mexico. *Food additives and contaminants, 20*(11), 1077-1086. DOI: https://doi.org/10.1080/02652030310001594478

42. Cassel, E. K., Campbell, B., Draper, M., & Epperson, B. (2012). Aflatoxin F907 Hazards in Grain Aflatoxicosis and Livestock. South Dakota State University Cooperation Extension Service/College of Agriculture and Biological Sciences/USDA. *Brookings, South Dalota, USA.*

43. Çelik, T. H., Sarımehmeto lu, B., & Küplülü, Ö. (2005). Aflatoxin $M_1$ contamination in pasteurised milk. *Veterinarski arhiv, 75*(1), 57-65. https://hrcak.srce.hr/67058

44. Chipley, J. R., & Uraih, N. (1980). Inhibition of **Aspergillus** growth and aflatoxin release by derivatives of benzoic acid. *Applied and Environmental Microbiology, 40*(2), 352-357. https://aem.asm.org/content/40/2/352.short

45. Chohan, A.S. (1983). Historical study of society and culture in Dardistan and Ladakh.

https://agris.fao.org/agris-search/search.do?recordID=US201300409315

46. Chohan, K. A., Awan, F., Ali, M. M., Iqbal, U., & Ijaz, M. (2016). Assessment of aflatoxin in dairy concentrate feeds, total mixed rations, silage and various feed ingredients in Pakistan. *Pakistan Journal of Zoology, 48*(1).

https://www.zsp.com.pk/pdf48/277280%20(35)%20Short%20communications%20QPJZ-0050-2015%2017-8-15.pdf

47. Choudhary, A. K. (1992). Influence of microbial co-inhabitants on aflatoxin synthesis of *Aspergillus flavus* on maize kernels. *Letters in applied microbiology, 14*(4), 143-147. DOI: https://doi.org/10.1111/j.1472-765X.1992.tb00670.x

48. Choudhary, A. K., & Kumari, P. (2010). Management of mycotoxin contamination in preharvest and post harvest crops: present status and future prospects. *Journal of Phytology*. 2(7), 37-52

http://updatepublishing.com/journal/index.php/jp/article/view/2160

49. Choudhary, A. K., & Sinha, K. K. (1993). Competition between a toxigenic Aspergillus flavus strain and other fungi on stored maize kernels. *Journal of Stored Products Research, 29*(1), 75-80. DOI: https://doi.org/10.1016/0022-474X(93)90025-Y

50. Choudhary, A. K., Kumari, P., & Aggarwal, R. (2014). RAPD based DNA fingerprinting of toxigenic and non-toxigenic strains of *Aspergillus flavus* isolated from different habitats. *Indian Phytopathology, 67*(3), 291-297.

51. Choudhary, A. K., Tudu, S., Kumari, P., & Ranjan, A. (2020). Present status, prevalence and seasonal variations of aflaxtoxin in cattle feed, Bihar, India. *Indian Journal of Science and Technology, 13*(17), 1738-1745. DOI: 10.17485/IJST/v13i17.288

52. Churchill, K. (2017). The carry-over of aflatoxins in dairy feed to milk of modern holstein dairy cows. Cornell University. DOI: https://doi.org/10.7298/X43R0R2S

53. Colak, H. (2007). Determination of aflatoxin $M_1$ levels in Turkish White and Kashar cheeses made of experimentally contaminated raw milk. *Journal of Food and Drug Analysis* 15, (2), 9.

54. Cole, R. J. (1986). Etiology of turkey —X|| disease in retrospect: a case for the involvement of cyclopiazonic acid. *Mycotoxin research, 2*(1), 3-7. DOI: https://doi.org/10.1007/BF03191956

55. Cooney, D.O. (1980). Activated Charcoal: antidotal and other medical uses. Marcel Dekker. Inc. New York, NY.

56. Costamagna, D., Gaggiotti, M., Chiericatti, C. A., Costabel, L., Audero, G. M. L., Taverna, M., & Signorini, M. L. (2019). Quantification of aflatoxin M1 carry-over rate from feed to soft cheese. *Toxicology reports, 6,* 782-787. DOI: https://doi.org/10.1016/j.toxrep.2019.07.004

57. Cotty, P. J., Egel, D. S., & Elias, K. S. (1994). Relationships among isolates of *Aspergillus* sect. Flavi that vary in aflatoxin production. *pathology, 84906,* 912.

58. Crisan, E. V. (1973). Effects of aflatoxin on seeding growth and ultrastructure in plants. *Applied Microbiology, 26*(6), 991-1000. https://aem.asm.org/content/26/6/991.short

59. Cucullu, A. F., Pons Jr, W. A., & Goldblatt, L. A. (1972). Fast screening method for detection of aflatoxin contamination in cottonseed products. *Journal of the Association of Official Analytical Chemists, 55*(5), 1114-1119. DOI:

https://doi.org/10.1093/jaoac/55.3.1114

60. Cupid, B. C., Lightfoot, T. J., Russell, D., Gant, S. J., Turner, P. C., Dingley, K. H., ... & Garner, R. C. (2004). The formation of $AFB_1$-macromolecular adducts in rats and humans at dietary levels of exposure. *Food and chemical toxicology, 42*(4), 559-569. DOI: https://doi.org/10.1016/j.fct.2003.10.015

61. Dashek, W. V., & Llewellyn, G. C. (1974). Influence of the carcinogen aflatoxin $B_1$ on the metabolism of germinating lily pollen. In *Proceedings International Symposium on Fertilization in Higher Plants*. https://agris.fao.org/agris-search/search.do?recordID=US201302737178

62. De Iongh, H., Vies, R. O. & van Pelt, J. G. (1964). Milk of mammals fed an aflatoxm-containmg diet. *Nature,* London. 202, 466. DOI: 10.1038/202466a0

63. Demeke, T., Kidane, Y., & Wyhib, E., (1979). Ergotism: a report of an epidemic, 1977–78. *Ethiopian Medical Journal 17,* 107–114.

64. Deveci, O. (2007). Changes in the concentration of aflatoxin $M_1$ during manufacture and storage of White Pickled cheese. *Food Control, 18*(9), 1103-1107. DOI: https://doi.org/10.1016/j.foodcont.2006.07.012

65. Diaz, G. J., & Murcia, H. W. (2011). Biotransformation of aflatoxin $B_1$ and its relationship with the differential toxicological response to aflatoxin in commercial poultry species. *Aflatoxins-Biochemistry and Molecular Biology, 1,* 3-20.

66. Diekman, M. A., & Green, M. L. (1992). Mycotoxins and reproduction in domestic livestock. *Journal of animal science, 70*(5), 1615-1627. DOI: https://doi.org/10.2527/1992.7051615x

67. Diener, U. L., Cole, R. J., Sanders, T. H., Payne, G. A., Lee, L. S., & Klich, M. A. (1987). Epidemiology of aflatoxin formation by *Aspergillus flavus*. *Annual review of phytopathology*, *25*(1), 249-270. https://www.annualreviews.org/doi/citedby/10.1146/annurev.py.25.090187.001341

68. Divakara, S. T., Aiyaz, M., Hariprasad, P., Nayaka, S. C., & Niranjana, S. R. (2014). *Aspergillus flavus* infection and aflatoxin contamination in sorghum seeds and their biological management. *Archives of Phytopathology and Plant Protection*, *47*(17), 2141-2156. DOI: https://doi.org/10.1080/03235408.2013.869892

69. Dowelmadina, I. M. M., El Zubeir, I. E. M., Salim, A. D. A., & Arabi, O. H. M. H. (2014). Global Journal of Animal Scientific Research. *Global Journal of Animal Scientific Research*, *2*(2), 120-129. http://citeseerx.ist.psu.edu/viewdoc/download?doi=10.1.1.674.3587&rep=rep1&type=pdf

70. Drobotko, V. G. E. (1974). Stachybotryotoxicosis. A new disease of horses and humans. *American Review of Soviet Medicine*, *2*(3), 238-42.

71. Duarte, S. C., Almeida, A. M., Teixeira, A. S., Pereira, A. L., Falcão, A. C., Pena, A., & Lino, C. M. (2013). Aflatoxin M1 in marketed milk in Portugal: Assessment of human and animal exposure. *Food Control*, *30*(2), 411-417.

DOI: https://doi.org/10.1016/j.foodcont.2012.08.002 202

72. Eaton, D. L., and Groopman, J.D., (1994). The Toxicology of Aflatoxins. Academic Press, New York, pp: 383-426

73. El-Nezami, H. S., Nicoletti, G., Neal, G. E., Donohue, D. C., & Ahokas, J. T. (1995). Aflatoxin $M_1$ in human breast milk samples from Victoria, Australia and Thailand. *Food and chemical toxicology*, *33*(3), 173-179. DOI: https://doi.org/10.1016/0278-6915(94)00130-G

74. Elzupir, A. O., & Elhussein, A. M. (2010). Determination of aflatoxin $M_1$ in dairy cattle milk in Khartoum State, Sudan. *Food control*, *21*(6), 945-946. DOI: https://doi.org/10.1016/j.foodcont.2009.11.013

75. Engel, G., & Teuber, M. (1990). Toxic metabolites from fungal cheese starter cultures (*Penicillium camemberti* and *Penicillium roqueforti*) In: Van Egmond HP, editor. Mycotoxins in dairy products. London: Elsevier applied science. pp 163–192.

76. Eskola, M., Kos, G., Elliott, C. T., Hajšlová, J., Mayar, S., & Krska, R. (2020). Worldwide contamination of food-crops with mycotoxins: Validity of the widely cited FAO estimate'of 25%. *Critical reviews in food science and nutrition*, *60*(16), 2773-2789. DOI: https://doi.org/10.1080/10408398.2019.1658570

77. Fallah, A. A. (2010). Assessment of aflatoxin M1 contamination in pasteurized and UHT milk marketed in central part of Iran. *Food and Chemical Toxicology*, *48*(3), 988-991. DOI: https://doi.org/10.1016/j.fct.2010.01.014

78. Fink-Gremmels, J. (2008). Mycotoxins in cattle feeds and carry-over to dairy milk: A review. *Food Additives and Contaminants, 25*(2), 172-180.

DOI: https://doi.org/10.1080/02652030701823142

79. Gabbai, A., Lisbonne., Pourquier, (1951). Ergot poisoning at Pont St. Esprit. British Medical Journal Sept, 15, 650-651. DOI: 10.1136/bmj.2.4732.650

80. Galvano, F., Galofaro, V., & Galvano, G. (1996). Occurrence and stability of aflatoxin M1 in milk and milk products: a worldwide review. *Journal of Food protection, 59*(10), 1079-1090.

DOI: https://doi.org/10.4315/0362-028X-59.10.1079

81. Galvano, F., Pietri, A., Bertuzzi, T., Fusconi, G., Galvano, M., Piva, A., & Piva, G. (1996). Reduction of carryover of aflatoxin from cow feed to milk by addition of activated carbons. *Journal of Food Protection, 59*(5), 551-554.

DOI: https://doi.org/10.4315/0362-028X-59.5.551

82. Ghanem, I., & Orfi, M. (2009). Aflatoxin M1 in raw, pasteurized and powdered milk available in the Syrian market. *Food Control, 20*(6), 603-605. DOI: https://doi.org/10.1016/j.foodcont.2008.08.018

83. Gnonlonfin, G. J. B., Adjovi, Y., Gbaguidi, F., Gbenou, J., Katerere, D., Brimer, L., & Sanni, A. (2011). Scopoletin in cassava products as an inhibitor of aflatoxin production. *Journal of Food Safety, 31*(4), 553-558. DOI: https://doi.org/10.1111/j.1745-4565.2011.00334.x

84. Gnonlonfin, G. J. B., Hell, K., Adjovi, Y., Fandohan, P., Koudande, D. O., Mensah, G. A., ... & Brimer, L. (2013). A review on aflatoxin contamination and its implications in the developing world: a sub-Saharan African perspective. *Critical reviews in food science and nutrition, 53*(4), 349-365. DOI: https://doi.org/10.1080/10408398.2010.535718

85. González-Hernández, J., Méndez-Albores, J. A., Arámbula-Villa, G., Loarca-Piña, M. G., Castaño-Tostado, E., & Moreno-Martınez, E. (2004). Aflatoxins' fate during the nixtamalization of contaminated maize by two tortilla-making processes. *Journal of stored products research, 40*(1), 87-94. DOI: https://doi.org/10.1016/S0022-474X(02)00080-2

86. Govaris, A., Roussi, V., Koidis, P. A., & Botsoglou, N. A. (2001). Distribution and stability of aflatoxin $M_1$ during processing, ripening and storage of Telemes cheese. *Food Additives & Contaminants, 18*(5), 437-443. DOI: https://doi.org/10.1080/02652030120550

87. Gqaleni, N., Smith, J. E., & Lacey, J. (1996). Co-production of aflatoxins and cyclopiazonic acid in isolates of *Aspergillus flavus*. *Food additives & contaminants, 13*(6), 677-685. DOI: https://doi.org/10.1080/02652039609374453

88. Gürbay, A., Engin, A. B., Ça layan, A., & ahin, G. (2006). Aflatoxin $M_1$ levels in commonly consumed cheese and yogurt samples in Ankara, Turkey. *Ecology of Food and Nutrition, 45*(6), 449-459. DOI: https://doi.org/10.1080/03670240600985274

89. Guthrie, L. D., & Bedell, D. M. (1979). Effects of aflatoxin in corn on production and reproduction in dairy cattle. In *Proceedings, annual meeting of the United States Animal Health Association* (No. 83, p. 202). https://pubmed.ncbi.nlm.nih.gov/298916/

90. Harrison, A. L., Taber, R. A., Schroeder, H. W., & Pettit, R. E., (1971). Influence of fungicides and irrigation practice on aflatoxin in peanuts before digging. *Applied microbiology, 22*(4), 629-634.

91. Harvey, R. B., Kubena, L. F., Elissalde, M. H., Corrier, D. E., Huff, W. E., Rottinghaus, G. E., & Clement, B. A. (1991). Cocontamination of swine diets by aflatoxin and diacetoxyscirpenol. *Journal of Veterinary Diagnostic Investigation, 3*(2), 155-160. DOI: https://doi.org/10.1177/104063879100300210

92. Hashemi, M. (2016). A survey of aflatoxin M1 in cow milk in Southern Iran. *Journal of food and drug analysis, 24*(4), 888-893. DOI: https://doi.org/10.1016/j.jfda.2016.05.002

93. Heinonen, J. T., Fisher, R., Brendel, K., & Eaton, D. L. (1996). Determination of Aflatoxin B1 Biotransformation and Binding to Hepatic Macromolecules in Human Precision Liver Slices. *Toxicology and applied pharmacology, 136*(1), 1-7. DOI: https://doi.org/10.1006/taap.1996.0001

94. Henry, S. H., & Cardwell, K. F. (2004). Risk of exposure to and mitigation of effect of aflatoxin on human health: a West African example. *Journal of Toxicology: Toxin Reviews, 23*(2-3), 217-247. DOI: https://doi.org/10.1081/TXR-200027817

95. Henry, S. H., Whitaker, T., Rabbani, I., Bowers, J., Park, D., Price, W., ... & Coker. (2001). Aflatoxin M. In: Safety evaluation of certain mycotoxins in food. Prepared by the fifty-sixth Meeting of the joint FAO/WHO expert Committee on food Additives (JECFA). FAO Food and nutirition paper No. 74 Rome (Italy): FAO of UN.

96. Hoffmann, V., Jones, K., & Leroy, J. (2015). Mitigating aflatoxin exposure to improve child growth in Eastern Kenya: study protocol for a randomized controlled trial. *Trials, 16*(1), 1-7. DOI: https://doi.org/10.1186/s13063-015-1064-8

97. Hussain, I., Anwar, J., Munawar, M. A., & Asi, M. R. (2008). Variation of levels of aflatoxin $M_1$ in raw milk from different localities in the central areas of Punjab, Pakistan. *Food Control, 19*(12), 1126-1129. DOI: https://doi.org/10.1016/j.foodcont.2007.12.002

98. Hussain, I., Anwar, J., Asi, M. R., Munawar, M. A., & Kashif, M. (2010). Aflatoxin $M_1$ contamination in milk from five dairy species in Pakistan. *Food control, 21*(2), 122-124.DOI: https://doi.org/10.1016/j.foodcont.2008.12.004

99. Huwig, A., Freimund, S., Käppeli, O., & Dutler, H. (2001). Mycotoxin detoxication of animal feed by different adsorbents. *Toxicology letters, 122*(2), 179-188. DOI: https://doi.org/10.1016/S0378-4274(01)00360-5

100. Ikawa, M., Ma, D. S., Meeker, G. B., & Davis, R. P. (1969). Use of Chlorella in mycotoxin and phycotoxin research. *Journal of Agricultural and Food Chemistry, 17*(3), 425-429. DOI: https://doi.org/10.1021/jf60163a044

101. Inglis, G. D., & Kawchuk, L. M. (2002). Comparative degradation of oomycete, ascomycete, and basidiomycete cell walls by mycoparasitic and biocontrol fungi. *Canadian Journal of Microbiology, 48*(1), 60-70. DOI: https://doi.org/10.1139/w01-130

102. Ismail, A., Riaz, M., Akhtar, S., Yoo, S. H., Park, S., Abid, M., ... & Ahmad, Z. (2017). Seasonal variation of aflatoxin $B_1$ content in dairy feed. *Journal of Animal and Feed Sciences, 26*(1), 33-37. DOI: 10.22358/jafs/69008/2017

103. Jacquet, M., Cukier-Kahn, R., Pla, J., & Gros, F. (1971). A thermostable protein factor acting on *in vitro* DNA transcription. *Biochemical and biophysical research communications, 45*(6), 1597-1607. DOI: https://doi.org/10.1016/0006-291X(71)90204-X

104. Jeswal, P., Sinha, R. K., & Prasad, T. (1987). Seed mycoflora of cereals and aflatoxin contamination under various storage systems. *Journal of the Indian Botanical Society, 66*(1-2), 156-160.

105. Johnson, G. T. & White, J. P., (1982). Aflatoxin production correlated with nitrification in *Aspergillus flavus* group species. *Mycologia, 74*(5), 718-723. DOI: https://doi.org/10.1080/00275514.1982.12021578

106. Jones, F. T., Wineland, M. J., Parsons, J. T., & Hagler Jr, W. M. (1996). Degradation of aflatoxin by poultry litter. *Poultry science, 75*(1), 52-58. DOI: https://doi.org/10.3382/ps.0750052

107. Kala , P. (2011). The effects of silage feeding on some sensory and health attributes of cow's milk: A review. *Food Chemistry, 125*(2), 307-317. DOI: https://doi.org/10.1016/j.foodchem.2010.08.077

108. Kaleibar, M. T., & Helan, J. A. (2013). A field outbreak of aflatoxicosis with high fatality rate in feedlot calves in Iran. *Comparative Clinical Pathology, 22*(6), 1155-1163. DOI: https://doi.org/10.1007/s00580-012-1543-1

109. Kamkar, A., Karim, G., Aliabadi, F. S., & Khaksar, R. (2008). Fate of aflatoxin $M_1$ in Iranian white cheese processing. *Food and Chemical Toxicology, 46*(6), 2236-2238. DOI: https://doi.org/10.1016/j.fct.2008.02.028

110. Kamkar, A., Yazdankhah, S., Mohammadi Nafchi, A., & Mozaffari Nejad, A. S. (2014). Aflatoxin $M_1$ in raw cow and buffalo milk in Shush city of

Iran. *Food Additives & Contaminants: Part B*, 7(1), 21-24. DOI: https://doi.org/10.1080/19393210.2013.830277

111. Kang, M. S. (1970). Pathogenesis in groundnut *(Arachis hypogaea L.) by Aspergillus flavus* Link ex Fries (Doctoral dissertation, Ph. D. Dissertation. College of Agriculture, Punjab Agricultural University, Ludhiana 96 pp).

112. Kanungo, L., Bacher, G., & Bhand, S. (2014). Flow-based impedimetric immunosensor for aflatoxin analysis in milk products. *Applied biochemistry and biotechnology*, *174*(3), 1157-1165. DOI: https://doi.org/10.1007/s12010-014-0995-y

113. Klich, M. A., & Pitt, J. I. (1986). The theory and practice of distinguishing species of the *Aspergillus flavus* group. In *Advances in Penicillium and Aspergillus systematics* (pp. 211-220). Springer, Boston, MA. DOI: https://doi.org/10.1007/978-1-4757-1856-0_19

114. Kos, J., Levi , J., uragi , O., Koki , B., & Miladinovi , I. (2014). Occurrence and estimation of aflatoxin M1 exposure in milk in Serbia. *Food Control*, *38*, 41-46. DOI: https://doi.org/10.1016/j.foodcont.2013.09.060

115. Kozakiewicz, Z., Highley, E., & Johnson, G. I. (1996). Occurrence and significance of storage fungi and associated mycotoxins in rice and cereal grains. *Mycotoxin contamination in grains*, Australian Center for International Agricultural Research Technical Report Series, 37: 18– 26.

116. Krishnamachari, K. A. V. R., & Bhat, R. V. (1976). Poisoning by ergoty bajra (pearl millet) in man. *Indian journal of medical research*, *64*(11), 1624-1628.

117. Krishnamurthy, Y. L., & Shashikala, J. (2006). Inhibition of aflatoxin B1 production of *Aspergillus flavus*, isolated from soybean seeds by certain natural plant products. *Letters in applied microbiology*, *43*(5), 469-474. DOI: https://doi.org/10.1111/j.1472-765X.2006.02011.x

118. Krstovi , S., Vranješ, A. P., Kasalica, A., Jevti , M., & Jaji , I. (2018). Aflatoxin $M_1$ Transfer Rate from Milk into Cheese and Whey During the Production of Hard Cheese. *Contemporary Agriculture*, *67*(3-4), 215-220. DOI: https://doi.org/10.1515/contagri-2018-0031

119. Kumari P. (2018) Studies on characterization and micro-sequencing of aflatoxin resistance associated protein of aflatoxin resistance associated protein (RAP) variability of *Aspergillus flavus*. *PhD Thesis*.

120. Kurtzman, C. P., Horn, B. W., & Hesseltine, C. W. (1987). *Aspergillus nomius*, a new aflatoxin-producing species related to *Aspergillus flavus* and *Aspergillus tamarii*. *Antonie van leeuwenhoek*, *53*(3), 147-158. DOI: https://doi.org/10.1007/BF00393843

121. Langat, G., Tetsuhiro, M., Gonoi, T., Matiru, V., & Bii, C. (2016). Aflatoxin $M_1$ contamination of milk and its products in Bomet County, Kenya. *Advances in Microbiology*, *6*(07), 528. DOI: 10.4236/aim.2016.67053

122. Le Bars, J., & Le Bars, P. (1979). Cyclopiazonic acid bioproduction by *Penicillium camemberti* Thom effect of temperature on individual strains. In *Anuales De Recherches Veterinaries* (Vol. 10, No. PP. 601-602)

123. Lee, H. J., & Ryu, D. (2017). Worldwide occurrence of mycotoxins in cereals and cereal-derived food products: public health perspectives of their co-occurrence. *Journal of Agricultural and Food Chemistry, 65*(33), 7034-7051. DOI: https://doi.org/10.1021/acs.jafc.6b04847

124. Lee, S. E., Mahoney, N. E., & Campbell, B. C. (2002). Inhibition of Aflatoxin $ B1 $ Biosynthesis by Piperlongumine Isolated from *Piper longum* L. *Journal of microbiology and biotechnology, 12*(4), 679-682. https://www.koreascience.or.kr/article/JAKO200211921170425.pdf

125. Lillehoj, E. B., Ciegler, A., & Hall, H. H. (1967). Aflatoxin B1 uptake by *Flavobacterium aurantiacum* and resulting toxic effects. *Journal of Bacteriology, 93*(1), 464-471. https://jb.asm.org/content/93/1/464.short

126. Lilly, L. J. (1965). Induction of chromosome aberrations by aflatoxin. *Nature, 207*(4995), 433-434. DOI: 10.1038/207433a0

127. Lizarraaga-Paulin, E. G., Torres-Pacheco, I., & Moreno-Martinez, E. Miranda-Castro, S.P. (2011). Chitosan application in maizeczea mays to counteract the effects of abiotic stress at reedling level. Africal Journal of Biotechnology, 10(3): 6439-6446.

128. Madali, B., Gulec, A., & Ayaz, A. (2018). A survey of Aflatoxin M1 in different milk types in Turkey: risk assessment of children's exposure. Prog. Nutr, 20, 659-664. DOI: 10.23751/pn.v20i4.6889

129. Magan N and Olsen M. (Eds.). (2004). *Mycotoxins in food: detection and control.* Woodhead Publishing, *Cambridge, England*, 406-409.

130. Malloy, C. D., & Marr, J. S. (1997). Mycotoxins and public health: a review. *Journal of public health management and practice: JPHMP, 3*(3), 61-69. DOI: 10.1097/00124784-199705000-00013

131. Manetta, A. C., Giammarco, M., Di Giuseppe, L., Fusaro, I., Gramenzi, A., Formigoni, A., ... & Lambertini, L. (2009). Distribution of aflatoxin M1 during Grana Padano cheese production from naturally contaminated milk. *Food Chemistry, 113*(2), 595-599. DOI: https://doi.org/10.1016/j.foodchem.2008.07.091

132. Marasas, W. F. O., Kriek, N. P. J., Wiggins, V. M., Steyn, P. S., Towers, D. K., & Hastie, T. J. (1979). Incidence, geographic distribution, and toxigenicity of *Fusarium* species in South African corn. *Phytopathology, 69*(11), 1181-1185. DOI: 10.1094/Phyto-69-1181

133. Marin, S., Ramos, A. J., Cano-Sancho, G., & Sanchis, V. (2013). Mycotoxins: Occurrence, toxicology, and exposure assessment. *Food and chemical toxicology, 60*, 218-237. DOI: https://doi.org/10.1016/j.fct.2013.07.047

134. Martins, H. M., Guerra, M. M. M., & Bernardo, F. M. D. A. (2007). Occurrence of aflatoxin B1 in dairy cow's feed over 10 years in Portugal. *Rev Iberoam Micol, 24*, 69-71. https://www.reviberoammicol.com/2007-24/069071.pdf

135. Masoero, F. R. A. N. C. E. S. C. O., Gallo, A., Moschini, M., Piva, G. I. A. N. F. R. A. N. C. O., & Diaz, D. (2007). Carryover of aflatoxin from feed to milk in dairy cows with low or high somatic cell counts. *Animal, 1*(9), 1344-1350. DOI: https://doi.org/10.1017/S1751731107000663

136. Mehan, V. K., Mayee, C. D., Jayanthi, S., & McDonald, D. (1991). Preharvest seed infection by *Aspergillus flavus* group fungi and subsequent aflatoxin contamination in groundnuts in relation to soil types. *Plant and Soil, 136*(2), 239-248. DOI: https://doi.org/10.1007/BF02150055

137. Michlig, N., Signorini, M., Gaggiotti, M., Chiericatti, C., Basílico, J. C., Repetti, M. R., & Beldoménico, H. R. (2016). Risk factors associated with the presence of aflatoxin M1 in raw bulk milk from Argentina. *Food Control, 64*, 151-156. DOI: https://doi.org/10.1016/j.foodcont.2015.12.025

138. Mitchell, N. J., Bowers, E., Hurburgh, C., & Wu, F. (2016). Potential economic losses to the US corn industry from aflatoxin contamination. *Food Additives & Contaminants: Part A, 33*(3), 540-550. DOI: https://doi.org/10.1080/19440049.2016.1138545

139. Mohammadi, H. (2011). A review of aflatoxin $M_1$, milk, and milk products. *Aflatoxins–biochemistry and molecular biology'.(Ed. DRG Guevara-Gonzalez) pp*, 397-414.

140. Mozafari, S., Mohsenzadeh, M., & Mehrzad, J. (2017). Seasonally feed-related aflatoxins B1 and M1 spread in semiarid industrial dairy herd and its deteriorating impacts on food and immunity. *Journal of Food Quality, 2017*. DOI: https://doi.org/10.1155/2017/4067989

141. Nile, S. H., Park, S. W., & Khobragade, C. N. (2016). Occurrence and analysis of aflatoxin M1 in milk produced by Indian dairy species. *Food and Agricultural Immunology, 27*(3), 358-366. DOI: https://doi.org/10.1080/09540105.2015.1104655

142. Nishimwe, K., Bowers, E., Ayabagabo, J. D. D., Habimana, R., Mutiga, S., & Maier, D. (2019). Assessment of aflatoxin and fumonisin contamination and associated risk factors in feed and feed ingredients in Rwanda. *Toxins, 11*(5), 270. DOI: https://doi.org/10.3390/toxins11050270

143. Nummi, M., Ml, N. P., & Tm, E. (1975). Effect of a Fusarium-Toxia on the development of alpha-amylase activity in germinating barley. https://pascalfrancis.inist.fr/vibad/index.php?action=getRecordDetail&idt=PASCAL7638000866

144. Obonyo, M. A., & Salano, E. N. (2018). Perennial and seasonal contamination of maize by aflatoxins in eastern Kenya. *International*

*Journal of Food Contamination*, *5*(1), 6. DOI: https://doi.org/10.1186/s40550-018-0069-y

145. Omeiza GK. (2019). Aflatoxin Risk in Dairy Production: Assessment of Dairy Cattle Feed Contamination Level by *Aspergillus Flavus* and *A. Parasiticus* in both Conventional and Traditional Dairies. *Global Journal of Medical Research*. 1(3). DOI: 10.21106/ijtmrph.V3.N1s

146. Oruc, H. H., Cibik, R., Yilmaz, E., & Kalkanli, O. (2006). Distribution and stability of aflatoxin M1 during processing and ripening of traditional white pickled cheese. *Food Additives and Contaminants*, *23*(2), 190-195. DOI: https://doi.org/10.1080/02652030500389048

147. Ostry, V., Malir, F., Toman, J., & Grosse, Y. (2017). Mycotoxins as human carcinogens—the IARC Monographs classification. *Mycotoxin research*, *33*(1), 65-73. DOI: https://doi.org/10.1007/s12550-016-0265-7

148. Packa, D. (1991). Cytogenetic changes in plant cells as influenced by mycotoxins. *Mycotoxin Research*, *7*(2), 150-155. DOI: https://doi.org/10.1007/BF03192201

149. Pandya, J. P., & Arade, P. C. (2016). Mycotoxin: a devil of human, animal and crop health. *Advances in Life Sciences*, *5(10)*, 3937-3941.

150. Papp, E., Klara, H., Záray, G., & Mincsovics, E. (2002). Liquid chromatographic determination of aflatoxins. *Microchemical journal*, *73*(1-2), 39-46. DOI: https://doi.org/10.1016/S0026-265X(02)00048-6

151. Paranagama, P. A., Abeysekera, K. H. T., Abeywickrama, K., & Nugaliyadde, L. (2003). Fungicidal and anti-aflatoxigenic effects of the essential oil of *Cymbopogon citratus* (DC.) Stapf.(lemongrass) against *Aspergillus flavus* Link. isolated from stored rice. *Letters in Applied Microbiology*, *37*(1), 86-90. DOI: https://doi.org/10.1046/j.1472-765X.2003.01351.x

152. Phillips, T. D., Pimpukdee, K. L. F. K., Kubena, L. F., Bailey, C. A., Huebner, H. J., & Afriyie-Gyawu, E., (2004). Aflatoxin-induced toxicity and depletion of hepatic vitamin A in young broiler chicks: Protection of chicks in the presence of low levels of NovaSil PLUS in the diet. *Poultry science*, *83*(5), 737-744. DOI: https://doi.org/10.1093/ps/83.5.737

153. Pleadin, J., Vuli , A., Perši, N., Škrivanko, M., Capek, B., & Cvetni , . (2015). Annual and regional variations of aflatoxin B1 levels seen in grains and feed coming from Croatian dairy farms over a 5-year period. *Food Control*, *47*, 221-225. DOI: 10.1016/j.foodcont.2014.07.017

154. Prandini, A., Tansini, G. I. N. O., Sigolo, S., Filippi, L. A. U. R. A., Laporta, M., & Piva, G. (2009). On the occurrence of aflatoxin M1 in milk and dairy products. *Food and chemical toxicology*, *47*(5), 984-991. DOI: 10.1016/j.fct.2007.10.005

155. Pratiwi, C., Rahayu, W. P., Lioe, H. N., Herawati, D., Broto, W., & Ambarwati, S. (2015). The effect of temperature and relative humidity for Aspergillus flavus BIO 2237 growth and aflatoxin production on soybeans. *International Food Research Journal, 22*(1), 82.

156. Price, R. L., Lough, O. G., & Brown, W. H. (1982). Ammoniation of whole cottonseed at atmospheric pressure and ambient temperature to reduce aflatoxin M1 in milk. *Journal of Food Protection, 45*(4), 341-344. DOI: https://doi.org/10.4315/0362-028X-45.4.341

157. Rahimi, E., Bonyadian, M., Rafei, M., & Kazemeini, H. R. (2010). Occurrence of aflatoxin $M_1$ in raw milk of five dairy species in Ahvaz, Iran. *Food and Chemical Toxicology, 48*(1), 129-131. DOI: https://doi.org/10.1016/j.fct.2009.09.028

158. Rama, A., Latifi, F., Bajraktari, D., & Ramadani, N. (2015). Assessment of aflatoxin M1 levels in pasteurized and UHT milk consumed in Prishtina, Kosovo. *Food Control, 57*, 351-354. DOI: https://doi.org/10.1016/j.foodcont.2015.04.021

159. Rao, B. L., & Husain, A. (1985). Presence of cyclopiazonic acid in kodo millet (*Paspalum scrobiculatum*) causing kodua poisoning'in man and its production by associated fungi. *Mycopathologia, 89*(3), 177-180. DOI: https://doi.org/10.1007/BF00447028

160. Rastogi, S., Dwivedi, P. D., Khanna, S. K., & Das, M. (2004). Detection of aflatoxin M1 contamination in milk and infant milk products from Indian markets by ELISA. *Food control, 15*(4), 287-290. DOI: https://doi.org/10.1016/S0956-7135(03)00078-1

161. Reddy, T. V., Viswanathan, L., & Venkitasubramanian, T. A. (1970). Thin-layer chromatography of aflatoxins. *Analytical Biochemistry, 38*(2), 568-571. DOI: 10.1016/0003-2697(70)90487-2

162. Reiss, J. (1978). Mycotoxins in foodstuffs. XI. Fate of aflatoxin B1 during preparation and baking of whole-meal wheat bread. *Pascal Francis*, 55 (4), 421-423. DOI: http://pascal-francis.inist.fr/vibad/index.php?action=getRecordDetail&idt=PASCAL7910102528

163. Robens, J. F., & Richard, J. L. (1992). Aflatoxins in animal and human health. In *Reviews of environmental contamination and toxicology* (pp. 69-94). Springer, New York, NY. DOI: https://doi.org/10.1007/978-1-4613-9751-9_3

164. Ruscito, A., Smith, M., Goudreau, D. N., & DeRosa, M. C. (2016). Current status and future prospects for aptamer-based mycotoxin detection. *Journal of AOAC International, 99*(4), 865-877. DOI: https://doi.org/10.5740/jaoacint.16-0114

165. Santini, A., Raiola, A., Ferrantelli, V., Giangrosso, G., Macaluso, A., Bognanno, M., ... & Ritieni, A. (2013). Aflatoxin M1 in raw, UHT milk and dairy products in Sicily (Italy). *Food Additives & Contaminants: Part B, 6*(3), 181-186. DOI: https://doi.org/10.1080/19393210.2013.780186

166. Sargeant, K., Sheridan, A., O'kelly, J., & Carnaghan, R. B. A. (1961). Toxicity associated with certain samples of groundnuts. *Nature, 192*(4807), 1096-1097. DOI: https://doi.org/10.1038/1921096a0

167. Sarkisov, A. H. (1954). Mycotoxicoses (fungal poisonings). *Mycotoxicoses (fungal poisonings).* https://www.cabdirect.org/cabdirect/abstract/19591302245

168. Sarma, U. P., Bhetaria, P. J., Devi, P., & Varma, A. (2017). Aflatoxins: implications on health. *Indian Journal of Clinical Biochemistry, 32*(2), 124-133. DOI: https://doi.org/10.1007/s12291-017-0649-2

169. Sawatzky, G. A., Van Der Woude, F., & Morrish, A. H. (1969). Mössbauer study of several ferrimagnetic spinels. *Physical Review, 187*(2), 747. DOI: https://doi.org/10.1103/PhysRev.187.747

170. Schoental, R., & White, A. F. (1965). Aflatoxins and'albinism'in plants. *Nature, London, 205*(4966), 57-58. https://www.cabdirect.org/cabdirect/abstract/19661301045

171. Setlem, K., Mondal, B., Ramlal, S., & Kingston, J. (2016). Immuno affinity SELEX for simple, rapid, and cost-effective aptamer enrichment and identification against aflatoxin $B_1$. *Frontiers in microbiology, 7*, 1909. DOI: https://doi.org/10.3389/fmicb.2016.01909

172. Shantha, T., & Sreenivasa Murthy, V. (1977). Photo-destruction of aflatoxin in groundnut oil. *Indian Journal of Technology, 15*(10), 453-454. DOI: http://ir.cftri.com/id/eprint/7018

173. Siddappa, V., Nanjegowda, D. K., & Viswanath, P. (2012). Occurrence of aflatoxin $M_1$ in some samples of UHT, raw & pasteurized milk from Indian states of Karnataka and Tamilnadu. *Food and chemical toxicology, 50*(11), 4158-4162. DOI: https://doi.org/10.1016/j.fct.2012.08.034

174. Sinha, K.K. & Bhatnagar D. (1997). Agricultural and Food Safety.

175. Sinha K.K. & Choudhary, A.K. (2008). Mycotoxins: Toxicity, Diagnosis Regulation and control through Biotechnology. *Annual Review of Mycology & plant pathology,* Vol. 4, Indian Society of Mycology and Plant Pathology, Scientific Publishers (India): Jodhpur pp. 261-299

176. Sinha, K.K. (1983). Aflatoxin problem in storage and standing maize crops. Mycotoxins in food and feed. Allied Press, India, 23-36.

177. Sinha, A. K., & Sinha, K. K. (1990). Insect pests, *Aspergillus flavus* and aflatoxin contamination in stored wheat: a survey at North

Bihar (India). *Journal of Stored Products Research, 26*(4), 223-226. DOI: 10.1016/0022-474X(90)90026-O

178. Sinha, K. K. (1987). Aflatoxin contamination of maize in flooded areas of Bhagalpur, India. *Applied and environmental microbiology, 53*(6), 1391-1393. https://aem.asm.org/content/53/6/1391.short

179. Sinha, K. K., & Kumari, P. (1989). Effect of ochratoxin A on some biochemical changes in seeds of mung bean (*Vigna radiata*, var Pusa 119. *Journal of the Science of Food and Agriculture, 48*(4), 453-457. DOI: https://doi.org/10.1002/jsfa.2740480407

180. Sinha, K. K., & Singh, A. (1982). Aflatoxin producing potentials of *Aspergillus flavus* and natural occurrences of aflatoxins in some fruits and vegetables. *National Academy Science Letters-India, 5*(7), 213-214.

181. Smith, E. E., Phillips, T. D., Ellis, J. A., Harvey, R. B., Kubena, L. F., Thompson, J., & Newton, G. (1994). Dietary hydrated sodium calcium aluminosilicate reduction of aflatoxin M1 residue in dairy goat milk and effects on milk production and components. *Journal of Animal Science, 72*(3), 677-682. DOI: https://doi.org/10.2527/1994.723677x

182. Smith, J. E., & Moss, M. O. (1985). *Mycotoxins. Formation, analysis and significance*. John Wiley & Sons Ltd. https://www.cabdirect.org/cabdirect/abstract/19861314084

183. Spesivtseva, N. A. (1960). Mycoses and mycotoxicoses of animals. *Mycoses and mycotoxicoses of animals*. https://www.cabdirect.org/cabdirect/abstract/19652202945

184. Stoev, S. D. (2013). Food safety and increasing hazard of mycotoxin occurrence in foods and feeds. *Critical reviews in food science and nutrition, 53*(9), 887-901.

DOI: https://doi.org/10.1080/10408398.2011.571800

185. Sullivan Jr, J. D., & Ikawa, M. (1972). Variations in inhibition of growth of five Chlorella strains by mycotoxins and other toxic substances. *Journal of agricultural and food chemistry, 20*(4), 921-922. DOI: https://doi.org/10.1021/jf60182a044

186. Tahoun, A. B., Ahmed, M. M., Abou Elez, R. M., & AbdEllatif, S. S. (2017). Aflatoxin $M_1$ in Milk and some Dairy Products: Level, Effect of Manufature and Public Health Concerns. *Zagazig Veterinary Journal, 45*(2), 188-196. DOI: 10.21608/ZVJZ.2017.7891

187. Tajkarimi, M., Aliabadi-Sh, F., Nejad, A. S., Poursoltani, H., Motallebi, A. A., & Mahdavi, H. (2008). Aflatoxin $M_1$ contamination in winter and summer milk in 14 states in Iran. *Food Control, 19*(11), 1033-1036. DOI: https://doi.org/10.1016/j.foodcont.2007.10.011

188. Thomas, F., Eppley, R. M., & Trucksess, M. W. (1975). Rapid screening method for aflatoxins and zearalenone in corn. *Journal of the Association of Official Analytical Chemists, 58*(1), 114-116. DOI: https://doi.org/10.1093/jaoac/58.1.114

189. Tripathi, R. K., & Misra, R. S. (1983). Mechanism of inhibition of maize seed germination by aflatoxin $B_1$. *Mycotoxins in Food and Feed*, 129-141.

190. Trucksess, M. W., Richard, J. L., Stoloff, L., McDonald, J. S., & Brumley, W. C. (1983). Absorption and distribution patterns of aflatoxicol and aflatoxins $B_1$ and $M_1$ in blood and milk of cows given aflatoxin $B_1$. *American Journal of Veterinary Research, 44*(9), 1753.

191. Ueno, Y. (1980). Trichothecene mycotoxins mycology, chemistry, and toxicology. In *Advances in nutritional research* (pp. 301-353). Springer, Boston, MA. DOI: https://doi.org/10.1007/978-1-4757-4448-4_10

192. Ullah, H. A., Durrani, A. Z., Ijaz, M., Javeed, A., Sadique, U., Hassan, Z. U., ... & Khattak, I. (2016). Dietary mycotoxins binders: A strategy to reduce aflatoxin M1 residues and improve milk quality of lactating Beetal goats. *Journal für Verbraucherschutz und Lebensmittelsicherheit, 11*(4), 305-309. DOI: https://doi.org/10.1007/s00003-016-1046-0

193. Uraguchi, K. (1971). Pharmacology of mycotoxins. *International encyclopedia of pharmacology and therapeutics*, 143-298.

194. Van der Fels-Klerx, H. J., Liu, C., & Battilani, P. (2016). Modelling climate change impacts on mycotoxin contamination. *World Mycotoxin Journal, 9*(5), 717-726. DOI: https://doi.org/10.3920/WMJ2016.2066

195. Van Egmond, H. P. (1994). *Aflatoxins in milk* (pp. 365-381). Academic Press, San Diego, CA.

196. Van Egmond, H. P., Svensson, U. K., & Fremy, J. M. (1997). Residues and contaminants in milk and milk products. *Mycotoxins. İnternational Dairy Federation Special*, (9701), 112.

197. Var, I., Erginkaya, Z., & Kabak, B. (2009). Reduction of ochratoxin A levels in white wine by yeast treatments. *Journal of the Institute of Brewing, 115*(1), 30-34. DOI: https://doi.org/10.1002/j.2050-0416.2009.tb00341.x

198. Veldman, A., Borggreve, G. J., Mulders, E. J., & Van de Lagemaat, D. (1992). Occurrence of the mycotoxins ochratoxin A, zearalenone and deoxynivalenol in feed components. *Food Additives & Contaminants, 9*(6), 647-655. DOI: https://doi.org/10.1080/02652039209374120

199. Virdis, S., Corgiolu, G., Scarano, C., Pilo, A. L., & De Santis, E. P. L. (2008). Occurrence of aflatoxin M1 in tank bulk goat milk and ripened goat cheese. *Food Control, 19*(1), 44-49. DOI: https://doi.org/10.1016/j.foodcont.2007.02.001

200. Völkel, I., Schröer-Merker, E., & Czerny, C. P. (2011). The carry-over of mycotoxins in products of animal origin with special regard to its implications for the European food safety legislation. *Food and Nutrition Sciences*, *2*(08), 852-867. DOI: : 10.4236/fns.2011.28117

201. Waliyar, F., Kumar, K. V. K., Diallo, M., Traore, A., Mangala, U. N., Upadhyaya, H. D., & Sudini, H. (2016). Resistance to pre-harvest aflatoxin contamination in ICRISAT's groundnut mini core collection. *European Journal of Plant Pathology*, *145*(4), 901-913. DOI: https://doi.org/10.1007/s10658-016-0879-9

202. Walte, H. G., Schwake-Anduschus, C., Geisen, R., & Fritsche, J. (2016). Aflatoxin: food chain transfer from feed to milk. DOI: https://doi.org/10.1007/s00003-016-1059-8

203. Williams, J. H. (2011). Aflatoxin as a public health factor in developing countries and its influence on HIV and other diseases. *Peanut Collaborative Research Support Program, University of Georgia, World Bank Report*, 1-95.

204. Wilson, D. M., & Payne, G. A. (1994). Factors affecting. *The toxicology of aflatoxins: Human health, veterinary, and agricultural significance.*

205. Wu, F. (2007). Measuring the economic impacts of **Fusarium** toxins in animal feeds. *Animal Feed Science and Technology*, *137*(3-4), 363-374. DOI: https://doi.org/10.1016/j.anifeedsci.2007.06.010

206. Wu, F., Bhatnagar, D., Bui-Klimke, T., Carbone, I., Hellmich, R., Munkvold, G., ... & Takle, E. (2011). Climate change impacts on mycotoxin risks in US maize. *World Mycotoxin Journal*, *4*(1), 79-93. DOI: 10.3920/WMJ2010.1246

207. Wu, F., Groopman, J. D., & Pestka, J. J. (2014). Public health impacts of foodborne mycotoxins. *Annual review of food science and technology*, *5*, 351-372. DOI: 10.1146/annurev-food-030713-092431

208. Wu, F., Shephard, G. S., & Khlangwiset, P. (2011). Aflatoxins and growth impairment: a review. *Critical reviews in toxicology*, *41*(9), 740-755. DOI: https://doi.org/10.3109/10408444.2011.575766

209. Wu, J., Zhou, Y., Yu, W., Xu, Y., Wang, P., Xie, B., & Chen, F. (2007). Preparation for aflatoxin $B_1$-cationized bovine serum albumin based on Mannich-type reaction. *Journal of immunological methods*, *328*(1-2), 79-88. DOI: https://doi.org/10.1016/j.jim.2007.08.009

210. Wu, L. S. F., Groopman, J. D., Egner, P. A., Schulze, K. J., Merrill, R., Mehra, S., ... & Khatry, S. K. (2014). Aflatoxin exposure during the first 1000 days of life in rural South Asia assessed by aflatoxin $B_1$-lysine albumin biomarkers. *Food and chemical toxicology*, *74*, 184-189. DOI: https://doi.org/10.1016/j.fct.2014.09.016

211. Yadagiri, B., & Tulpule, P. G. (1974). Aflatoxin in buffalo milk. *Indian journal of dairy science*. https://agris.fao.org/agris-search/search.do?recordID=US201303096372

212. Yousef, A. E., & Marth, E. H. (1989). Stability and degradation of aflatoxin $M_1$. *Mycotoxins in dairy products*, 127-161.

213. Zheng, N., Sun, P., Wang, J. Q., Zhen, Y. P., Han, R. W., & Xu, X. M. (2013). Occurrence of aflatoxin M1 in UHT milk and pasteurized milk in China market. *Food Control, 29*(1), 198-201. DOI: https://doi.org/10.1016/j.foodcont.2012.06.020

# COLOUR PLATES

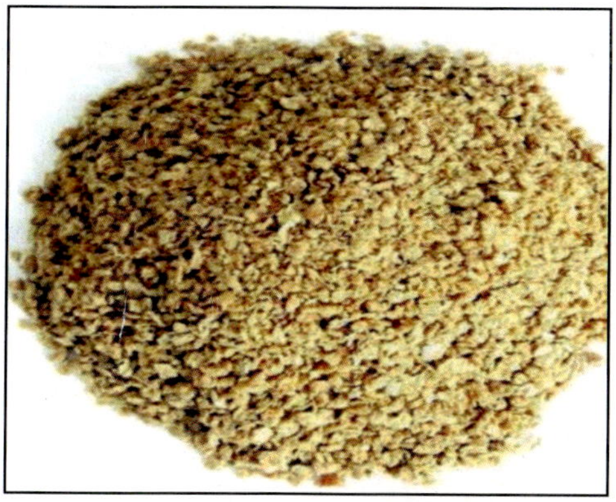

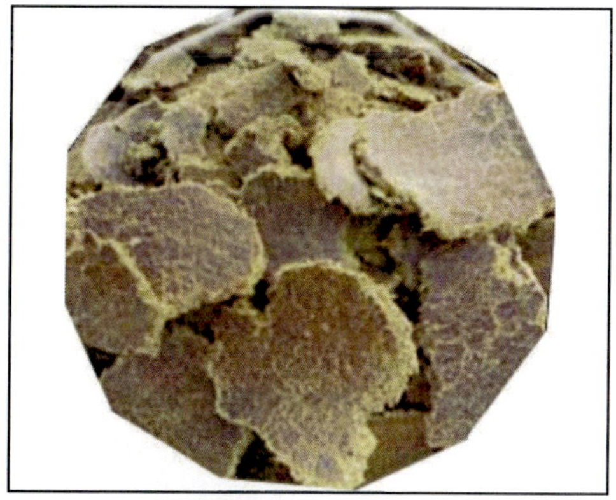

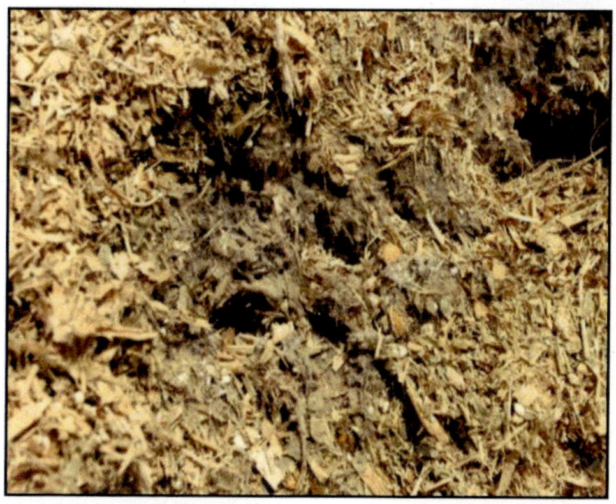

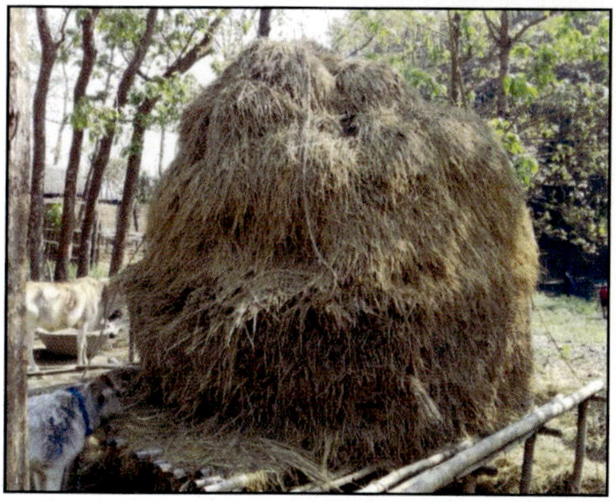

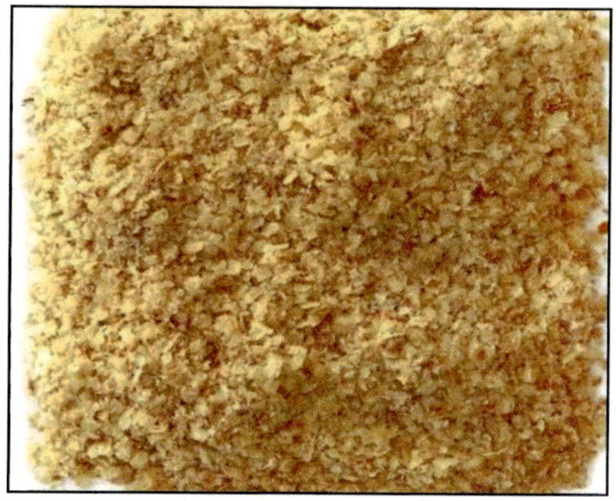

**(Types of Cattle Feed)**

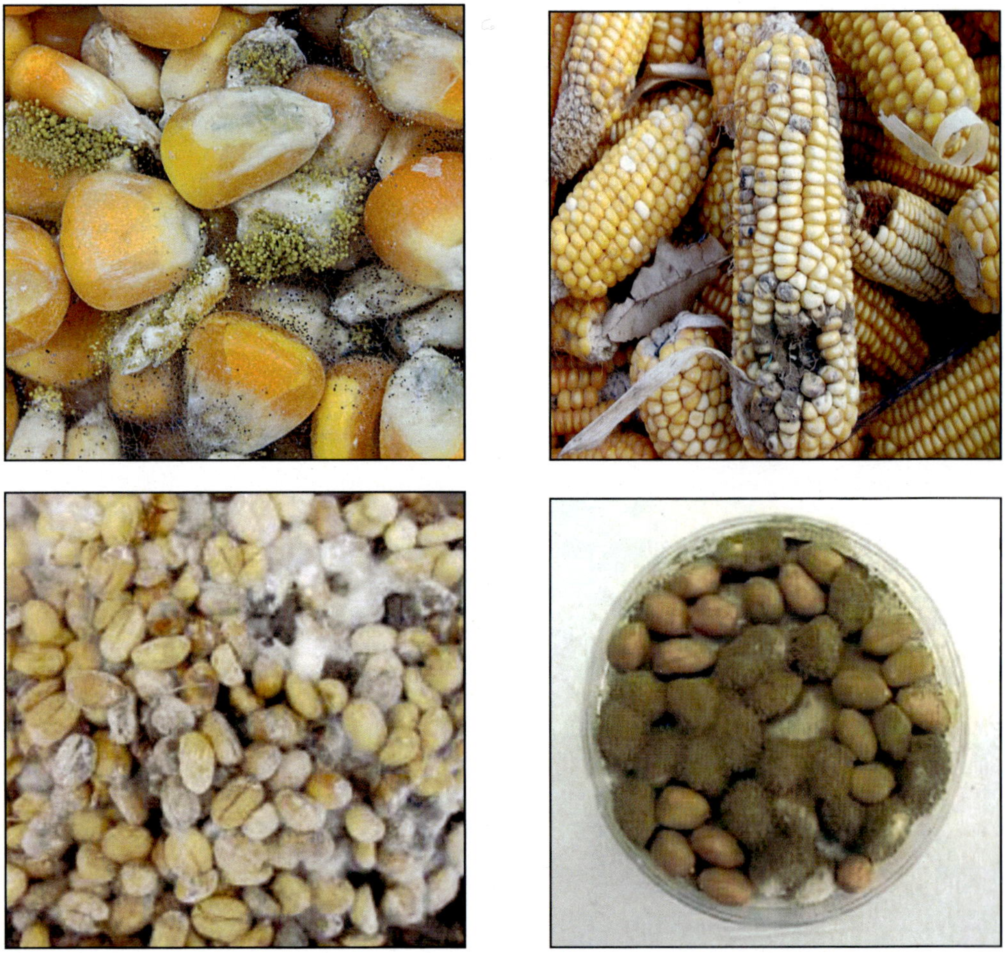

**(Contaminated Cattle Feed)**

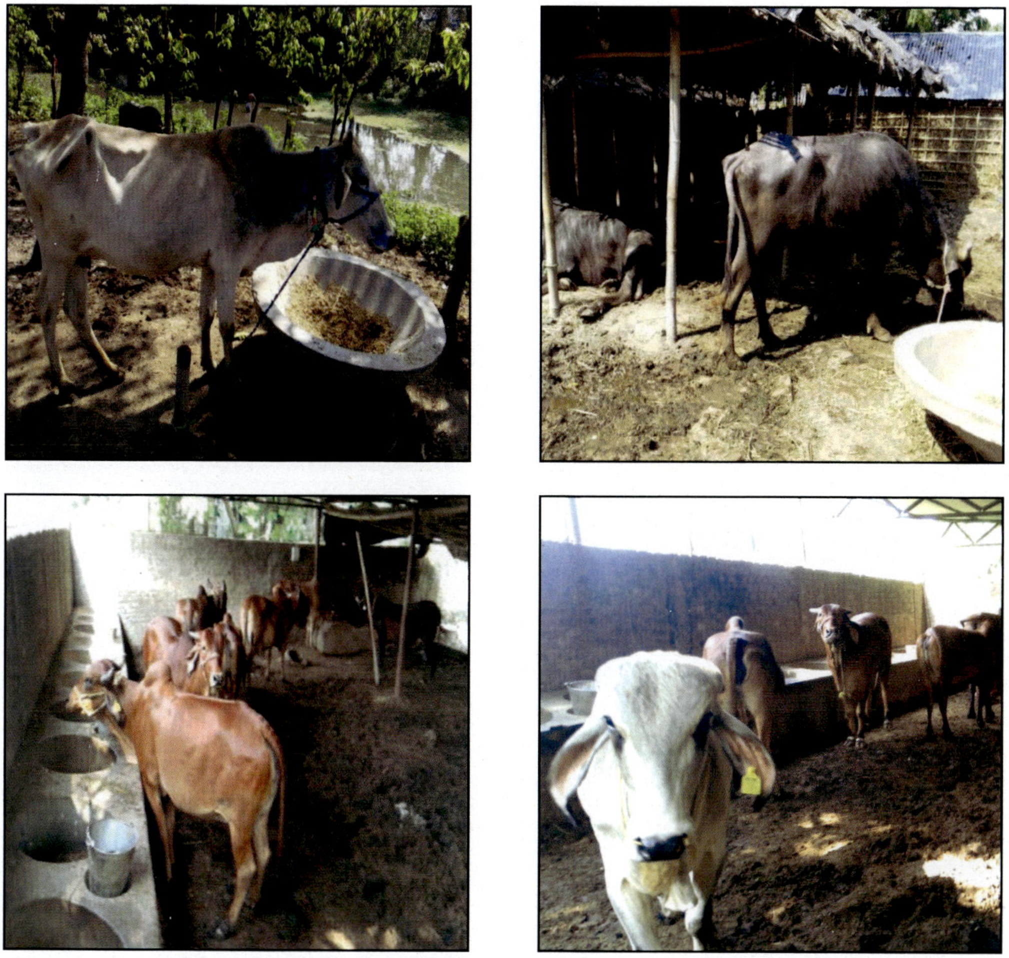

**(Cattle in Farm and in Rural Areas)**

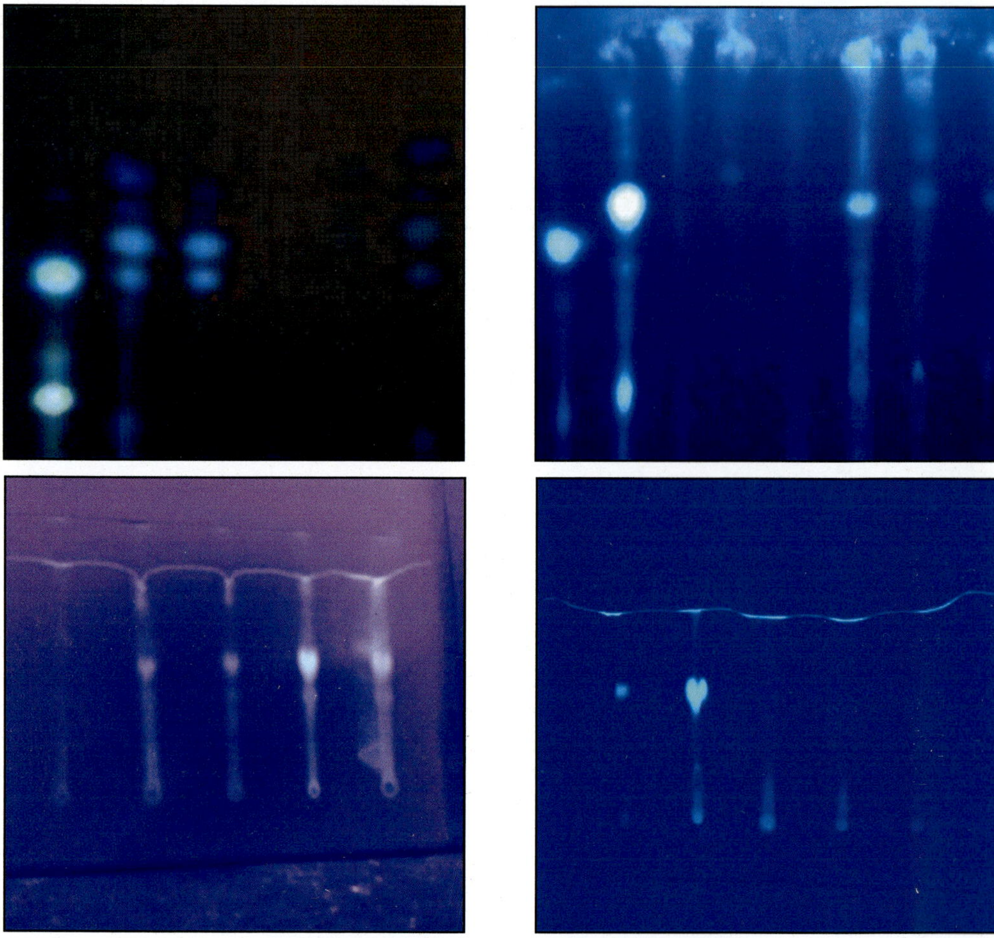

**(Aflatoxin B1 in TLC Plate)**

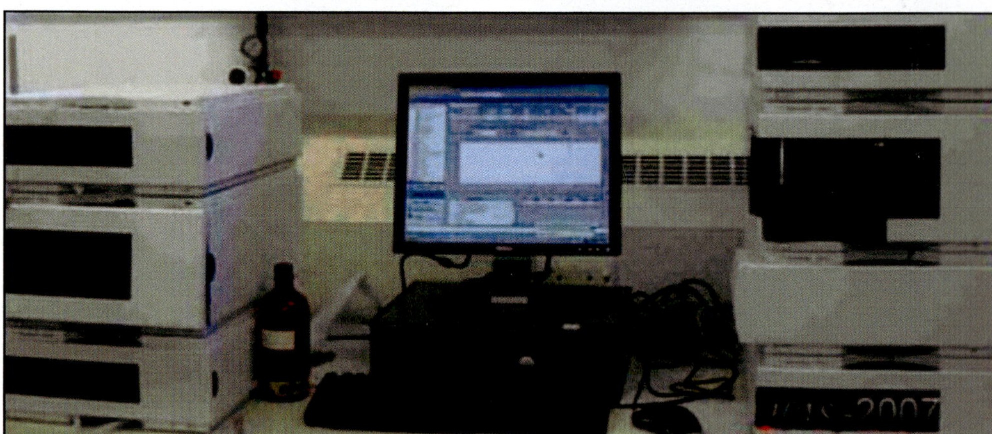

**(HPLC Apparatus for Aflatoxin Estimation)**

# INDEX